Professional ethics
and organisational change
in education and health

Professional ethics and organisational change in education and health

Edited by
Christine Henry

Professor of Applied Ethics and Head of the Centre for Professional Ethics, University of Central Lancashire, Preston, UK

Assistant Editor
Jane Pritchard

Edward Arnold
A member of the Hodder Headline Group
LONDON   MELBOURNE   AUCKLAND

First published in Great Britain 1995 by
Edward Arnold, a division of Hodder Headline PLC,
338 Euston Road, London NW1 3BH

Whilst the advice and information in this book is believed to be true and
accurate at the date of going to press, neither the author nor the publisher
can accept any legal responsibility or liability for any errors or omissions
that may be made.

British Library Cataloguing in Publication Data
A catalogue record for this book is available from the British Library

ISBN 0 340 60142 6 (Pb)

1 2 3 4 5   95 96 97 98

Typeset in 10/11pt Times by Phoenix Photosetting, Chatham, Kent
Printed and bound in Great Britain by J.W. Arrowsmith Ltd, Bristol

Acknowledgements

The editor and contributing authors would like to thank Louise Williams for her patience and tenacity throughout the writing of this book. The skills involved in the efficiency of word-processing often go unnoticed, where hours of work and continued moral support during the production and rearrangement of the text for publication provide an invaluable contribution. In addition, the list of contributors would be incomplete without acknowledgement of both the exceptionally gifted cartoonist, Wendy Michallat and technical editor, Catherine Cookson. Their contribution and skills are of equal importance in raising the profile, clarity and understanding of the text.

315676

Contents

Contributors

Julie Apps has a background in nursing education, applied ethics and psychology and is now studying for a PhD in Ethics and Psychology. She is a nurse tutor in Manchester and has published a significant number of articles in the health and nursing field.

George Campbell has a professional background in education. His academic development and interests are in English, cultural studies and applied ethics in higher education. He lectures in English literature as well as working part-time at the Centre for Professional Ethics on research.

Janine Drew has a professional background in diverse areas of administration. Her academic development and interests are in English literature, ethics and management practice within organisations. She is currently studying for her MPhil/PhD in ethics and management.

Norma Fryer has a professional background in nursing and midwifery education and management. She has recently completed a Masters degree in Health Care Ethics and now lectures in midwifery studies and ethics at the University of Central Lancashire. She is departmental co-ordinator for research. She has recently published articles and chapters in journals and texts.

Christine Henry has a professional background in health, psychology and education. Her academic development and interests are in the areas of philosophy, ethics and psychology specifically related to the professional fields of education, health research and management. She is Professor of Applied Ethics and Head of the Centre for Professional Ethics, University of Central Lancashire. She has substantial publications in various journals and books.

Mairi Levitt has a background in teaching in higher education. She has recently completed her PhD in Sociology and joined the Centre for Professional Ethics in 1993, to carry out research in the field of theology and education.

Glenys Pashley has a background in health psychology and philosophy and research for health and social work professionals. She has a Masters in business administration as well as one in psychology and education. She currently lectures in the Department of Social Work at the University of Central Lancashire. She has published articles and chapters in various journals and texts.

Jane Pritchard has a background in philosophy and has been a practising solicitor for several years. She joined the Centre for Professional Ethics in August 1993 as research assistant. Jane is currently involved with publications and conference presentations and assists Chris Henry with one of the centre's major research projects on professional conduct and codes. She is studying for a PhD.

Alan Roff has a background in quantitative social science and business information technology. He has published, taught and researched in these fields. He is currently Vice Rector of the University of Central Lancashire and has responsibility for all academic, research, commercial and international matters.

Margaret Yeomans has a background in nursing and midwifery and has both practised and taught in these fields.

Cartoonist

Wendy Michallat has a background in French, publishing and administration. She is currently reading for a Masters degree at Nottingham University. She is a cartoonist and has published in several magazines and newspapers as well as being commissioned by the Centre for Professional Ethics to do a series of cartoons for lectures and conferences.

Technical editor

Catherine Cookson taught English for many years in comprehensive schools and was Head of English at Prestwich High School, Bury. She is presently teaching English as a foreign language. She has been on the editorial board for the *Journal of Advances in Health Care*, Quay Publishing, Lancaster and has acted as technical editor on various books and publications.

Preface

This book evolved, in part, from the first Ethics and Values Audit carried out in a university in the UK. It should be identified as the first serious attempt in practical ethics to focus specifically upon 'people' organisations. The Ethics and Values Audit (abbreviated to EVA) was an in-house research based audit commissioned by the Rector of the University. A full summary of the EVA is explained, with a preface written by the Vice Rector of the University, in Appendix 2. The EVA is an attempt to synthesise theoretical and empirical enquiry aimed to provide further evidence for the development of a relationship between ethical theory and practice. As the co-ordinator of the research based audit, I have subsequently been stretched beyond the boundaries of academia into the realms of ethical reality and everyday morality within the organisational framework. My belief is that progress could not have been made with contemporary ethics without some evidence of first hand experience, particularly in times of rapid organisational change. The diversity of experience of my own and other contributors to the book has led to this first serious attempt at clarifying the importance of applied ethics. Although the book is essentially a work in practical ethics, where its foundation is within the organisational context, it has at its core the beginning of a search for a theoretical framework useful for solving practical problems. The book itself does not make a claim to have achieved this but at least attempts in some small way to contribute to the beginning of an ongoing process of enquiry introduced more specifically through professional ethics.

Professor John Wilcox, Director of the Centre for Professional Ethics at Manhattan College, New York, first introduced the idea of a value audit to the University on his visit in 1991. His contribution as an advisor for the first EVA project and his ongoing support for the project was acknowledged in 1993 when he was awarded the title of Honorary Professor in the Centre for Professional Ethics at the University of Central Lancashire. In part, the outcome of the first EVA saw the University develop and resource what is now a research centre for professional ethics. All the contributors of the book are in some way connected to the Centre either as members of staff, as members and advisors to the EVA project team itself or as professionals, social scientists and applied philosophers who are currently studying for their doctorate in applied ethics. The Centre for Professional Ethics has two professors, two research assistants, a senior lecturer, two administrators, two visiting professors and seven visiting fellows. Ruth Chadwick has recently joined the Centre as Professor of Moral Philosophy, enhancing the Centre's expertise in theoretical moral philosophy and

Bioethics. The Centre is in its infancy but hopefully may be seen to join others on the 'cutting edge' of applied ethics. All members have expertise in their own fields as well as a commitment to national and international 'networking'. Collaboration and the exchange and sharing of ideas are essential to encourage and facilitate the development of an ongoing process of ethical enquiry that may in turn contribute to better understanding of practical ethics. I thank all the contributors, advisors, supporters and publishers for their commitment to this first endeavour.

Christine Henry
University of Central Lancashire
Preston, Lancashire
UK

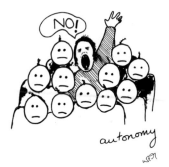

autonomy

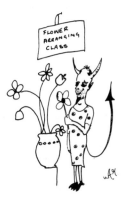

Non - maleficence

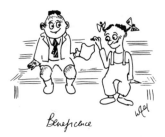

Beneficence

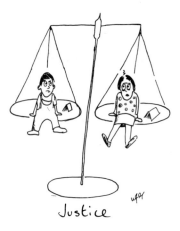

Justice

The Ethical Principles

Introduction

If we meet and do not agree, then perhaps we may still part as friends. If we pass on the street and do not speak perhaps we may at least smile. The world is both feeling and thought and if the stars are watching I would hope in a moral universe they may see us as friends!

The Ethics and Values Audit (EVA) carried out in 1992 was essentially an exploratory study of an organisation's ethical profile, from which this book was developed. The text is arranged into three sections in an attempt to develop a critique that follows a logical process of enquiry. The purpose of the book is to heighten the awareness of those ethical principles and values underpinning the management of organisational change. Furthermore, the book raises issues that seek to explore the type of ethical system needed to enhance a changing corporate culture. The chapters address some of the problems that arise within 'people organisations' identifying the need for a consensus of values and shared practices with an emphasis on developing a credible ethical theoretical framework from which these practices may be applied.

Section One identifies a framework from which the process of carrying out an ethics and values audit may be discussed.

Chapter 1 introduces and attempts to clarify some of the traditional moral principles and values formulating the essence of applied or professional ethics as a discipline of moral philosophy where clarification within the practical, organisational field is essential. The chapter also summarises selectively two major ethical theories, those of utilitarianism and Kantian duty ethics, in an attempt to identify their usefulness in solving moral conflict.

Chapter 2 examines and discusses change and common principles and values in relation to organisations within the health field. The discussion centres around issues and problems that arise when ideological, political and social factors impose their influence upon organisations and the members of the professional community. Chapter 3 highlights some of the ambiguity in the general interpretation of language, relating this in some way to the effect of language used within organisations and through applied ethics.

Section Two relates to the construction and application of EVA where different perspectives within the education and health field are addressed.

Chapter 4 introduces the implementation of the EVA and broadly identifies the relationship of the process of carrying out an audit with the development of mission statements, charters and codes. Chapter 5 takes the perspective further and examines and debates the audit process in terms of management and organisational change. Chapters 6 and 7 provide a brief summary of the EVA's findings relating the usefulness as a process to both the educational institutions in general and to those organisations where education and service are provided within the health sector.

Section Three consolidates the thematic development of empirical enquiry as a useful 'tool' for professional and organisational ethics.

Chapter 8 introduces social conceptions, values and principles underpinning equal opportunities and the organisation's policy. The chapter specifically explores the evolving relationship between ethical practice and the reality of equal opportunities. Chapter 9 identifies issues where there is a 'mismatch' of policy and practice. Utilising the EVA itself through a case study approach, it explores possibilities for development of an ethical system for managing change within the organisation. Chapter 10 develops the theme of professional ethics and explores in some depth a major moral principle in terms of organisational perceptions. This is discussed in terms of practice and introduces, within the practical context, an ethics of care.

The two appendices are equally important as part of the text, in that they not only identify the difficulties of ownership of values and forms of assessment but provide an honest and open summary of the first organisational ethics and values audit carried out within the United Kingdom.

In one sense the book defends a rational idealism within moral theory but hopes to exemplify the usefulness of traditional rational principles as essential for practical application. Whilst we shall always encounter and seek to resolve moral dilemmas, there appears to be a clear and necessary requirement to move from theory to practice in order to reach an appropriate place to meet. Our scientific enquiry is in its adolescent stage; *morally*, I would suggest we have been suspended in the womb! Perhaps the time of birth has arrived.

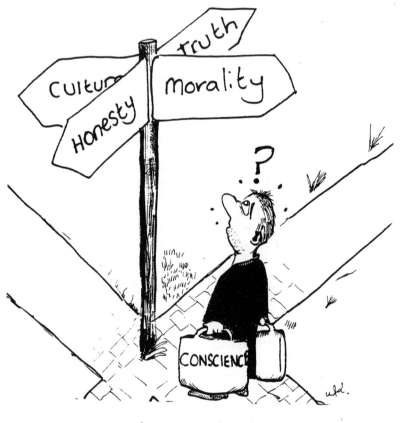

Ethical Conflict.

Section One
Theory and practice

1 Introduction to professional ethics for health care professionals

Christine Henry

This chapter examines professional ethics within the organisational framework. The author explores how principles and shared professional and organisational values are inherent and necessary for good practice. There is a discussion of how ethical analysis and synthesis may inform effective decision making and subsequently action within a changing organisational framework.

Echo was a nymph who did not take kindly to the god Pan's advances. In revenge he made the local shepherds mad. The shepherds tore poor Echo to pieces, and only her voice remained! However, she had a Voice. *'Ethics' – the echo heard always within the professional soul!*

Professional ethics

Accountability is central to professional practice within the organisational field. Gray and Pratt (1989) claim that personal accountability and ethical decision making are linked closely to what it is to be a professional. Being accountable involves taking responsibility for one's actions and decisions and is important for the setting of standards and norms. Furthermore, an organisation is collectively accountable for establishing and maintaining the standards of practice; for example an educational organisation's purpose involves high standards of learning and an health care organisation a high quality of care. Therefore it follows that there ought to be shared professional and organisational principles and values underpinning professional practice and the organisation's mission. It is necessary to discuss in some detail what we mean by principles and values.

Principles and values

Midgley (1991) remarks that applied ethics and morality relate to the whole of life within both our private and public domain. Ethics involves acting upon what we decide and by consequence, how we behave. Moral rules are central to ethical practice and the development of a caring community.It is therefore important to have a clear understanding of what constitutes moral principles and values. The term 'a caring community' may be applied to both health and educational organisations.

Principles are guidelines for human conduct that have a broad universal application and are central to the ways in which we behave towards each other. The principle of 'respect for persons' involves the action of positively caring and valuing other individuals and will always have implications for professional communities within the NHS and higher education.

> Most western, principle-based ethical systems have long tended to consider respect for persons a central and indispensable normative principle in moral reasoning
>
> (Keyserlingk, 1993, p390)

Respect for persons is one of the central principles underpinning professional practice. Henry and Pashley (1990) support Abelson's (1977) view that the term 'person' itself is a value-laden term like the moral term 'good'. Henry (1986), in her study of the concept of 'persons', states that the term 'person' is unanalysable and that it is impossible to define a 'person' by simply identifying intrinsic features or criteria such as having the ability to be rational, to communicate or to be self reflective. Abelson's view is supported where it seems that the term 'person' is a value term and features or criteria or specific behaviour will not give clear direction on who should and should not be defined as a person. A notable contemporary philosopher, Gilbert Ryle clearly stated that very young infants and idiots (his words) are not persons!

However, if the term 'person' is used like a moral term then it follows that *respect* for persons is an important moral principle inherent in professional practice. Respect involves valuing the person even though their own personal autonomy may be impaired and they cannot make choices without help; for example the very young infant requires an adult to act as advocate. Respect for persons as a central principle relates to other principles such as autonomy, non-maleficence, beneficence and justice. It is useful to attempt to show how these other moral principles relate to respect for persons simply because of their central role in professional ethics, health care and educational practice.

Personal *autonomy* is taken to mean being capable of making choices, being self-determined, responsible and capable of independent judgement without being constrained by some other person's action. Nevertheless, the term cannot be given a definition since it is value-laden and an ideal abstract term. It is obvious that the common cold can impair our autonomy. Usually in suffering from a cold our concentration is impaired and possibly our abilities to make clear decisions. It is therefore reasonable to assume that if people are seriously in need of health care their autonomy may be impaired. A common sense view informs us that any kind of emotional, psychological, social or physical disturbance will interfere with our personal autonomy. However, having personal autonomy relates to being a person and capable of making decisions and choices, *being an active not a passive soul without an echo*! It follows that if the term 'person' is a moral term like the term 'good' and *respect* for persons is maintained even if the person has lost the capacity to function in a self-determined way, likewise it is reasonable to claim respect for an individual's autonomy even if his/her autonomy is impaired. Some, but not all philosophers support the notion of respect for autonomy as being important for health care practice and it is often seen as important for education. If autonomy is taken to mean not just an intrinsic criterion/feature or trait for personhood but a moral principle, a value term like the concept of the person itself, then respect for persons and by consequence respect for personal autonomy follows. However, respect can only have sensibility through action and the way in which we behave towards each other.

It is reasonable to assume that the same principles of personal autonomy can apply to professional autonomy. Professional groups ought to be self-regulating and, through critical self-appraisal within the profession, be capable of maintaining some degree of professional autonomy. In this sense we may include educators, health care practitioners and managers in the professional cluster. No one profession will achieve absolute professional autonomy, although some professions, notably medicine and law, have traditionally been seen to have stronger professional autonomy than others. Sharing knowledge, ways of delivering care, team work and shared values and principles, together with valuing what each profession may give, will certainly improve professional practice and perhaps encourage respect for both personal and professional autonomy. What is needed is a more comprehensive interprofessional understanding of principles and values and the underpinning ethical framework.

Non-maleficence means to do no harm. This principle directly refers to not inflicting harm on others and implies action in this sense rather than being just a virtue or motive (Beauchamp and Childress, 1979). If this principle is not upheld harm may result through restriction of liberty by not having the freedom to make choices. The principle requires the individual to take due care not to inflict harm on others. It relates to the principle of respect for persons in that to do no harm may not only emphasise valuing others but avoids harming a person by restriction of liberty or autonomy. The principle of *beneficence* is more positive than non-maleficence because it requires that we ought to take positive action in order to help other persons, for example to positively care for others. Beneficence is important to the health care professions in that the professional may become an advocate for the patient or client who may have impaired autonomy through illness. However, beneficence is also important for the educator in positively doing good for the student. Beneficence, in the same way as non-maleficence, supports the principle of respect for autonomy and by consequence respect for persons. However, beneficence may conflict with autonomy. For example the professional may act in the best interest of the client/patient in order to avoid harm but the action may interfere with the client's wishes, values or beliefs. Some forms of treatment may be life-saving but the patient may refuse treatment; this is where legal processes apply. An educator may likewise act in the best interests of the student but this may also militate against the student's wishes, values and beliefs.

Justice is linked with the principle of respect for persons and governs the interactions between individuals or groups. The notion of fairness and equity is implicit in justice and it governs what is due and to whom. When justice is applied to organisations it ought to lead to informed decisions concerning the welfare of staff and clients. The concept of justice relates to policies such as equal opportunities and issues of what is right and just in the allocation of limited resources. Implicit within the meaning and application of these principles is an 'ethics of care' that specifically concerns action within a given context (see Chapter 10).

With person status go rights, responsibilities and respect for personal autonomy. If respect for persons is not both the focus and guiding principle to the professional codes and organisational goals, then it follows that the individual will be disadvantaged. We are all aware from social history the consequences of a race of people who had their person status taken from them along with its attendant rights, responsibilities and social identity. When individuals are not treated as persons or valued as persons, unethical practices occur. Within the organisation, an individual may be perceived by some only as a 'cost unit'. This example may be oversimplified, but serves to remind us of what can and does happen if principles are not in any sense used as guidelines.

Values

The learning of values apply to all educational systems and never more so than those who teach the professionals. MacIntyre (1987) remarks that the distinction between values that are both intrinsic and extrinsic to a social organisation is important for our understanding of moral problems. Thinking carefully about what sort of future changes we would want cannot be separated from examining our present values. Values are much more subjective than principles and are not necessarily moral. Some organisational values may conflict with professional or personal values. Values have a personal interpretation; they can violate or support principles. Wilcox and Ebbs (1992) remark that when institutions look towards a form of self-assessment they are required to assess progress through a commonly held bench-mark. This bench-mark is articulated through the mission or value system. However, in relation to substantiating a professionally ethical driven system, the values that are shared in both professional and organisational terms, must support moral principles. 'Values encompass not only morality but political, social, economic and aesthetic aspects of life' (Henry *et al.*, 1992 p32). Values may also be narrowly perceived and there is little doubt that Hitler had some very clear values that he imposed upon a whole nation. Values are central to a society's culture, attitudes and behaviour, involving individual personalities as well as groups. 'They flow from basic assumptions or world views, are the wellspring of the moral life and deeply influence ethical enquiry of that life' (Henry *et al.*, 1992, p109).

Whilst values embrace a diversity, in commonsense everyday language values and morals are juxtaposed. The notion of valuing actually encapsulates the idea of both knowing and doing. It is self-evident that moral values and the process of valuing concern thought and action and the notion of self-reflection provides the impetus for ethical analysis and debate. Ethics by definition assesses the ways in which we behave and those values that we possess. Personal and organisational life, guided by shared values and moral strategies will empower and affirm members of the organisation's community. However, it is worth remembering that a balance is required in that: 'While it is a truism that the unexamined life is not worth living, the life that is constantly under the microscope of ethical analysis in order to catch immorality will not be worth living either' (Henry *et al.*, 1992, p110).

Ethics, normative and professional

Morality refers to human conduct and values whereas ethics refers to the study of those. Common sense dictates that the two terms are used interchangeably However, morals may be perceived as prescriptions or rules to guide our actions and behaviour whereas ethics may be perceived as a set of analytical tools or a process that helps to identify right conduct and determine appropriate behaviour. In one sense morality is what we ideally aim for whereas ethics is a process that has a theoretical reflective and normative element that helps to achieve the aim. In other words the use of moral or ethical theory can be applied to help resolve dilemmas. Furthermore, ethics may be perceived as not only a process or tool but the outcome of analytical and moral enquiry.

Normative ethics is clearly a practical discipline dealing with practical moral problems (Edel, 1986). *Professional ethics* is derived from normative ethics and is applied to practical problems within an organisational and professional framework. Professional ethics is much more than a set of rules, codes or specified conduct formulated and enforced by the professions. Professional ethics involves reflective investigation that weighs up alternatives, uses ethical and theoretical application and adheres to the standards that reflect major ethical principles such as respect for persons. In other words, professional ethics is not just the construction of codes of professional practice developed by the professions, but in the widest and deepest sense involves normative enquiry and will employ appropriate theoretical application in an attempt to solve moral dilemmas. (It is perhaps important to remember that codes, missions or charters cannot solve moral dilemmas but they do have other important functions (see Chapters 2 and 5).) A set of identified rules of conduct founded upon the discipline of ethics is only part of the function of professional ethics. Furthermore, professional ethics, whilst clearly concerned with and applied to professional behaviour, hence its usefulness as an underpinning ethical framework for organisations, ought not to be seen as separate from mainstream ethics. When a person assumes a professional role, he/she automatically adopts moral responsibilities which may be perceived as more explicit than ordinary morality. This may occur when one is a member of a particular organisation or a specific profession, especially if there is an organisational code as well as codes for particular professions.

There is no obligation to become a nurse, doctor, educator or manager but the adopted role will nevertheless, clearly involve the person becoming accountable for the decisions taken and by consequence the action that follows. It is therefore essential to encourage better understanding and confidence in practical ethics. Professional ethics in the widest and deepest sense cuts across the specific disciplines and professions. Professional ethics may be perceived as encompassing a variety of specific professions such as medicine, nursing, business, management, education, law, science, technology and theology within its boundaries. This means that education of the professionals must involve ethical theory useful for practice. It is perhaps essential that our universities teach professional ethics as well as technical competence. Furthermore, professionals are directly involved on a day-to-day basis with specific ethical issues and therefore will bring useful insight and experience to the ethical problems encountered.

The application of ethics may be seen within any organisation and perhaps a brief summary of two major ethical theories may serve to emphasise the requirement for providing a synthesis of ethical approaches useful for practical application.

Utilitarianism

The major philosophers who developed the Utilitarian approach were Jeremy Bentham (1748–1832) and John Stuart Mill (1806–1873). Utilitarianism is the moral /ethical theory that states that right actions ought to produce the greatest happiness for the greatest number of people. Happiness is equated with good therefore the interpretation may be the maximum good for the greatest number of people. Utilitarianism takes the view that all knowledge comes from experience (empiricism). Whether an act is right or not depends on the consequences of an act. The situation or context is important and emphasis is given to the action, not to any generalised rule. There is an element of subjectivism in that the act of telling a lie may be right for one person and not for another. In this sense the theory is relative to the agent and the social context. What is moral is dependent upon the act and not on the motives of the agent. It is, therefore, perfectly acceptable for an organisation to give to charity in order to avoid paying high taxes. A good end will always justify the means and this reflects social utility. The theory is teleological in that it emphasises purpose as a way or means towards achieving happiness. Morality is created by a contract and things that are good or bad originate in society, not in the individual. Social utility emphasises that the general good is more important than individual rights and the principle of beneficence is pursued in order to positively help others in need. According to the utilitarians humans are not the only sentient beings that ought to be valued; other species feel pleasure and happiness and therefore have intrinsic value.

Criticism of utilitarianism

The major consequentialist theory of utilitarianism is not without its problems and whilst it may be useful for application in some conflicting situations, it does not help in others. Not only is there a difficulty in equating happiness with goodness; there is the problem of taking into account the total number of effects before an action can be assessed as right or wrong. We can never indisputably count the future consequences of an action. Furthermore we cannot measure in any sensible way the amount of pleasure over pain. Other philosophers would claim that the means cannot justify the ends and if we take a utilitarian view how do we find the best specific rule? For example 'a person known to be innocent should never be found guilty'. The utilitarian theory, whilst claiming that intention and a sense of duty are not the only criteria for moral worth, still avoids consideration of moral principles that are not based upon consequences, such as justice and fairness. Furthermore, should conduct be evaluated by considering the agent's motives? An organisational utilitarian position may deem an organisational policy, decision or action to be good, if it promotes the general welfare of the greatest number of people. Nevertheless, some actions may be inappropriate even if they produce the greater good. Suppose a policy is developed that avoids redundancy. In times of crisis individuals are reallocated to different roles in different departments to maximise the use of staff resources. The community benefits from this, in that security of employment for the majority is maintained. However, the individual is disadvantaged even if the consequences of reallocation benefit the common good. A minority of individuals may be unable to function well or even may show signs of incompetence due to the allocation of a specific role for which they are not trained. This in turn may do harm to the individual through loss of self-esteem and confidence. The consequences of such an action are impossible to predict.

Duty ethics

Duty ethics involves applying the same rule for everyone in all circumstances. Immanuel Kant (1724–1804) was the main proponent of duty ethics and made the assumption that all knowledge comes through the process of reason; the rightness or wrongness is determined by motives or duty. The consequences are irrelevant and if someone conforms or assents to a moral rule he/she must act accordingly. The context of a situation is quite irrelevant in that the rules apply to everyone: in this sense the theory is universal in that it prescribes the same moral rules to everyone no matter what the situation or circumstances. Rules are prior to action and the morality of the act is deduced from the rules. The theory is objective in that the rule is viewed as universal and independent of the agent. A Kantian perspective would insist that one should never lie regardless of the situation or circumstances. Absolute universal moral rules must be adhered to and the motives of the agent are considered important. Achieving a good end will never justify the means, therefore a deontological position is taken, in that abiding by the moral rules, having obligation and duty is seen as an end itself. The person is an end in him/herself and respect for persons is central. An organisation which gives to charity in order to avoid paying more taxes, even though the end is good, will be perceived as wrong. The Kantian view upholds private and individual morality and self-respect. The person has free will and is a moral agent, therefore morality derives from the individual and good and evil originate from human nature itself, not from society. The mind of the person is viewed as ontologically superior to the body. Life is an end in itself and therefore valuable, regardless of the quality; therefore the sanctity of human life is absolute. Justice and fairness are maintained and supportive of respect for persons and their autonomy.

Criticism of Kantian ethics

It may be the case that in everyday commonsense practice we do not
adhere to either theory in absolute terms but attempt a synthesis and
take what is useful from both approaches. Kantian ethics does not
handle cases where we have a conflict of duties. If one makes a promise
to keep a secret and then someone else asks you to tell the truth you
cannot do both. An absolute dictate from the Kantian perspective
would ask you to do both, yet it is impossible to universalise the
behaviour. Furthermore, the individual agent may be mistaken in
what constitutes a duty and thus act accordingly and do something
which is morally wrong. Alternatively, a person without any thought of
or idea of doing his duty may act in a moral way. It seems rather absurd
to deny them moral goodness. The claim that Kant makes never to tell
a lie is much too strong, in that there may be circumstances in which a
person cannot tell the truth because he is morally obligated not to do
so, in order to prevent harm. Moral rules are generalisations and
telling the truth and keeping promises should perhaps be adhered to if
there are no overriding factors evident. Suppose within your organisation a colleague tells you he is suffering from a chronic illness but asks
you to keep it a secret because his employment status would be
endangered. If you also recognise that his work is deteriorating and
others may suffer what do you do? In this sense personal moral values
may conflict with organisational values. The emphasis is upon the
individual, rather than consequences and the common good.

A synthesis

Moral dilemmas arise in every area of our lives; in the organisation in
which we work and in the professional areas of politics, education,
health, medicine, business and science. Whilst social scientists teach
descriptive ethics, philosophers continue to teach analytical and theoretical ethics. It is now necessary to derive a new synthesis in order to
address the real practical problems that modern society and its subsequent dynamic changes impose upon us. Moral education within the
professional and managerial areas of the universities must in some way
be encouraged and enhanced. In times of change how we deal with
moral values is reflected through the culture of the organisation. We
can no longer take the view that theory and practice within the ethical
domain are independent from each other. There is some necessity to
examine carefully whether *we practise what we preach* and look
towards ways in which there can be a synthesis of empirical, theoretical
and normative enquiry that underpins and formulates methods that
are ethically consistent and efficient in helping us solve our problems.
The aim is to produce the mature professional moral agent who not

only is aware of the ethical efficacy but can advocate an ethical system that will help to improve quality of practice and, in turn, better care. Traditional prescriptive ethics cannot, on its own, account for our experience of moral dilemmas and there is a need for a new synthesis in order to produce a more unified applicable ethical system that will enrich not only our moral development but our better understanding of practising what we preach!

Whilst any organisation will be influenced to some extent by external forces they are also shaped by the internal forces (Tierney, 1988). A culture of an organisation will be reflected in its achievements. Exploring the community, individual and group values give not only a picture of an organisation's culture but also a profile of what the potential development for that organisation might be. Covey (1989) suggests that values are maps that emerge from experience and have a subjective interpretative reality, alternatively principles are guidelines to human conduct with some enduring moral values. Principles are essential to ethical theory and provide standards for behaviour.

Ethics as a discipline is seen as part of theoretical enquiry within the philosophical field but it is also part of everyday commonsense in that, through interaction with others, individuals make certain choices. Ethics offers ways of enquiry into behaviour and gives justification for actions taken based upon those choices. Professional ethics is within the field of normative ethics and, more importantly, must lay down the foundations for a synthesis of empirical, theoretical and normative enquiry. Within both public and private organisations members of the community will be mainly concerned with professional issues, whether they are members of a specific profession or organisational network. Understanding through application of ethical theory may help resolve conflict. A moral dilemma occurs when an individual has to choose between two competing goods. For example, one may act in the best interest of staff or clients and the organisation but such action may militate against one's own best interest. The professional or manager may act in the best interest of the organisation but may find herself in conflict with her own personal values.

Conflicting obligations to employees and clients may pull the organisation in different directions. A synthesis of applying ethical theories may result in a commonsense morality. However, 'Common sense is not always the most reliable guide for sound moral principles'. (Henry *et al.*, p114).

Whilst it is very difficult to resolve moral dilemmas even through applying moral theory, *identification* of conflicting obligations in aspects of fairness and respect for persons is of paramount importance. Furthermore raising levels of ethical awareness and what constitutes good practice is essential for both the professional person and the organisation. Charters, mission statements and codes will not solve moral dilemmas but one of their functions involves raising levels of ethical awareness and hopefully encouraging ethical practice. Beyerstein (1993) remarks that codes serve important functions and that moral dilemmas can often be resolved by recourse to moral theory.

The stronger the ethos is in ethical values within the culture of an institution, the more distinctive the institution will appear
(Henry *et al.*, 1992, p123)

Conclusion

According to DeMarco and Fox (1986), everyone theorises about values and it is not limited to discussions between moral philosophers. Often disciplines other than philosophy will use moral theories of one kind or another to justify their own activities and try to resolve the problems within their own professional field. Members of the organisation's community, including the managers, are not exempt from this form of activity. In fact, it is essential in everyday management practice.

Professional ethics encompasses principles and values central to normative enquiry. It is clear that ethical issues arise in areas of management and professional decision making and involve individuals at all levels within the organisation. Any leader within an organisation is constantly under pressure from social, economic and ideological forces and, increasingly, organisations have a requirement to respond to these social pressures. There is constant concern for fair resource allocation, identifying priorities and informed decision making, which will have many influences directly affecting the members of the organisation's community. Ethical practice must permeate through the organisational values and management ethos.

References

Abelson, R. (1977) *Persons: A Study in Philosophical Psychology.* Macmillan, London.

Beauchamp, T.L. and Childress, J.F. (1979) *Principles of Biomedical Ethics.* Oxford University Press, Oxford.

Bellah, R.N., Madsen, R., Sullivan, W.M. *et al.* (1985) *Habits of the Heart: Individualism and Commitment to American Life.* Berkeley University Press, California.

Beyerstein, D. (1993) *The Functions and Limitations of Professional Codes of Ethics.* In *Applied Ethics; A Reader,* E.R. Winkler, J.R. Coombes (eds), pp.416–25. Blackwell Scientific Publications, Oxford.

Covey, S. (1989) *The Seven Habits of Highly Effective People: Restoring the Character Ethic*. Simon and Schuster, New York.

DeMarco, J.P. and Fox, M. (1986) *New Directions in Ethics: The Challenge of Applied Ethics*. Routledge and Kegan Paul, London, pp.1–20.

Edel (1986). Ethical Theory and Moral Practice; on the terms of their relation. In *New Directions in Ethics*, DeMarco, J.P., Fox, R.M. (eds), pp.317–35. Routledge and Kegan Paul, London.

Henry, C. (1986) *Conceptions of the Nature of Persons*. Unpublished PhD, Leeds University.

Henry, C. and Pashley, G. (1990) *Health Ethics*. Quay Publishers, Lancaster.

Henry, C., Drew, J., Anwar, N., Campbell, G. and Benoit-Asselman, D. (1992) *EVA Project: The Ethics and Values Audit*. University of Central Lancashire, Preston.

Keyserlingk, E.W. (1993) *Ethics, Codes and Guidelines for Health Care and Research: Can Respect for Autonomy be a Multi-cultural Principle?* In *Applied Ethics; A Reader*, E.R. Winkler, J.R. Coombs (eds), pp.390–415. Blackwell Scientific Publications, Oxford.

MacIntyre, A. (1987). *After Virtue a Study in Moral Theory*, second edition. Duckworth, London.

Midgley, M. (1991) *Wisdom, Information and Wonder*. Routledge, London.

Pratt, R. (1989) *Issues in Australian Nursing 2*. Churchill Livingstone, Edinburgh.

Tierney, W.G. (1988) Organisational culture in higher education: defining the essentials. *Journal of Higher Education*, **59(1)** 2–21.

Wilcox, J.R. and Ebbs, S.L. (1992) *The Leadership Compass: Values and Ethics in Higher Education*. George Washington University, Washington DC.

Editor's note to Chapter 2

Chapter 1 has introduced the reader to professional ethics and given an indication of its scope and application to organisations involved in change. As it is inappropriate in this essentially practical volume to go into ethical theory in detail, a brief outline has been provided of the two most popular theories, namely Kantian deontology and utilitarianism. The ethical principles are shown to be the 'tools of the trade', whereby professional ethics is able to put abstract theory into practice.

Chapter 2 will illustrate the assertions of Chapter 1 in relation to the living example of an organisation undergoing change exemplified by the National Health Service. The chapter identifies some political ideological portrayals of the ethical theories operating in practice and applies some of the ethical principles. There is a brief reference to professional codes with some implied comment on their usefulness or otherwise, as a means whereby the principles can become operative in the everyday work of health professionals.

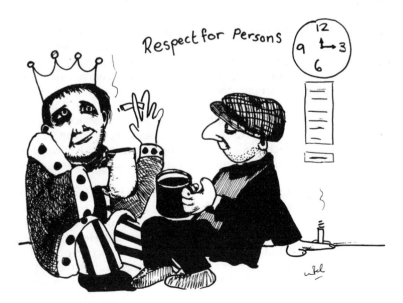

2 Applied ethics and managing change in the health field

Jane Pritchard

Introduction

The Conservative government of more than the last decade has dedicatedly pursued a campaign of deregulation of public utilities. The NHS is no exception to that endeavour. The theory which provides the rationale for this initiative would seem to fall between a Kantian promotion of individual autonomy with a minimum of (long-term) interference from the state and a sharing of resources between the largest number of people in a utilitarian bid to promote the least harm, if not the greatest good. Through 'boom' years and recession this programme has been pursued. Both sides of the political spectrum in this country would seem now to believe that the process is irreversible so, 'like it or lump it', it is incumbent upon us to understand the new structures and relationships and somehow make the best of it.

With the passing of the NHS and Community Care Act 1990 (HMSO, 1990a), the process of deregulation or 'privatisation' was begun. The management and structure of the NHS has been provided with a mechanism whereby the complete structure will be uprooted as the 'reforms' are phased in. Likewise legislation has played an important role in transforming the education of *health professional schooling*. Earlier years anticipated this change but without doubt, the present time is one of ongoing upheaval. With the introduction of new physical structures the government is prescribing a change in the psychological approach of all personnel operating in the health fields, be they in medicine, nursing, midwifery, para-medicine, management or health education.

The NHS finds its most dramatic change in the transition from state owned and state run units to independently financed and managed hospitals and doctors' surgeries. Health professional schooling has changed gradually since the Nurses, Midwives and Health Visitors Acts (HMSO, 1979 and 1992) that took away the function of training from the local health authorities and gave higher education the responsibility of providing education to degree level and beyond for health professionals.

These two very important structural changes strike at the heart of the management ethos required for the effective organisation of the

new service providers and the changed relationship with the purchasers of services. Formerly absent from public sector estab-
lishments, profit and competition are now firmly embedded in both
institution and personnel operating in these areas.

With the introduction of these two new concepts comes a whole new
psychological package for all levels of personnel employed by the
changed areas. The transformation is most apparent in the clinical
areas with the setting up of NHS trusts and GP Fundholders but is
nevertheless equally present in health education.

It has already been shown in Chapter 1 that such far reaching organisational change is likely to bring with it dangerous pitfalls for the institution if change is not introduced in a way that is firmly based on sound
and shared values. It will be shown that such values must be grounded
in ethical theory and wholly endorsed by all the people working in the
organisation. The discoveries of the EVA Report can be applied
equally to the changing health field as to higher education generally.

This chapter intends to identify the nature of the changes that have
taken place and which are still happening: change has and will occur on
an ongoing basis, each unit being reconstituted individually, particularly with regard to NHS trusts and GP fundholders. It will then discuss
the effect of change on the personality of the relevant institution and
the consequential psychological make-up of the new environment.
Using the EVA Report as a model it can be seen that there are
common areas of operation and its comment on practical ways of putting in place ethical foundations is identified as being advisable if
organisational change is to escape unnecessary and harmful pitfalls.

Definitions

This section will outline the meaning of the terms used in the context of
this chapter.

Health professionals means nurses, midwives, health visitors and
paramedics.
Health professional schooling means the training and/or education of
nurses, midwives, health visitors and paramedics.
Training means the training of health professionals as formerly provided within the health authorities.
Education means the education of health professionals as provided by
the higher education sector.
Providers means the providers of health services under the NHS and
Community Care Act 1990, namely NHS trusts and/or GP fundholders
and by extension, the providers of educational courses in higher
education.
Purchasers has the same meaning as in the NHS and Community Care

Act 1990 and briefly means the purchasers of health services, namely the local health authorities or the private sector and by extension, the health professional students.

Profit means the surplus (or shortfall) of income after the deduction of costs and is a sum in relation to the disposal of which the provider has freedom (subject to any statutory or other restraints).

Competition means the provision of services other than to a captive market, namely the provision of health services to purchasers pursuant to freely negotiated contracts and not by right or statutory requirement.

NHS trusts has the same meaning as in the NHS and Community Care Act 1990 and briefly means a hospital owned and run by a board of directors and not by a health authority.

GP fundholders has the same meaning as in the NHS and Community Care Act 1990 and briefly means a doctors' practice that is owned and run by the doctors and not directly funded or otherwise by a health authority or other statutory body.

Values has the same meaning as in the EVA Report and briefly means the broad bases or rules governing human conduct.

Ethical has the same meaning as in the EVA Report and, unlike values, refers to a 'good' motive governing human conduct.

EVA Report means the Ethics and Values Audit carried out in the University of Central Lancashire in 1992 and published as the EVA Project.

The legal structure of the NHS

The NHS and Community Care Act 1990 is the means whereby change occurs. It enables the establishment of NHS trusts and GP fundholders and specifies the new relationship that exists between these new animals, the local health authorities and the Department of Health. The role of the health authorities changes from being primarily responsible for the provision of medical care in the community to being the purchasers of services from NHS trusts to enable them to discharge their statutory obligation to supply identified local medical needs.

The devolution to NHS trusts of the ownership and control of hospital buildings and the function of employer to the managerial boards is a fundamental change. With ownership of assets, of course, go the answerability and responsibility for what happens to those assets. There is no proposal that there should be a change in the free treatment at the point of delivery policy. Thus the patient, whilst renamed in the Patient's Charter (HMSO, 1992) as client, is not the customer or purchaser of services. The purchaser of services from the NHS trust provider is the local health authority. Private patients or their insurance companies are also purchasers of services.

To govern the provision and purchase of services the local health authority enters into 'NHS contracts', that is, formal written agreements with NHS trusts setting the terms and standards whereby services will be provided. There is a statutory prohibition against undercutting the cost of services provided by units that continue to be state owned and run although if NHS trusts derive an unforeseen income from private sources that profit can be used to reduce the cost of providing services to the NHS patient. It is not clear exactly what this means but it would seem to give some scope for 'special offers' during the course of a trust's accounting year. Via the contract the trust earns the income necessary to provide health care services, employ staff, etc. and to maintain the loan payments, usually to the government. The loan of course was obtained by the trust in order to buy the buildings, equipment, staff, etc. when the trust was set up. The Chief Executive has a primary responsibility to ensure that the loan is repaid and that the trust remains financially viable.

Unless and until all hospitals and doctors' practices are 'privately' run there continues within the health authorities responsibility for the remaining units. The Government would seem to support entire devolution to trusts, however.

> Furthermore health authorities will want to concentrate on their role as purchasers of health services. It will be increasingly anomalous for them also to manage provider units.
>
> (HMSO, 1990b, p3)

The board of directors of an NHS trust consists of a non-executive chairman appointed by the Secretary of State and thereafter up to five non-executive directors and an equal number, including the Chief Executive and the Finance Director, of executive directors. It is likely that there will be a Clinical Director and a Nursing Director.

Day-to-day management structures are arranged by the Chief Executive who is responsible to the Board. Interestingly, directors are not personally liable for the actions of the board. Thus it could be argued that, as a legal entity the NHS trust is more akin to a limited company registered under the Companies' Acts than to a trust constituted under the Trustee Acts. Personal liability is a feature of a trustee but not generally of a company director. Of course the vast sums of money involved and responsibility for compensation claims in negligence actions would make a directorship extremely unattractive if personal liability was attached.

Arguably the absence of personal liability could reduce the commitment to the trust of senior management. From both an ethical and a legal standpoint there may be a greater risk to the patient receiving treatment from a trust as the chain of liability stops with the finite assets of the individual trust, rather than the larger health authority, as was formerly the case. As I am not privy to NHS contracts that are privately negotiated, it is impossible to say whether any residual liability vests with the local authority. If there were a major disaster, however, where a trust was guilty of gross negligence resulting in a large number of patients being awarded compensation, then the possibility should be noted that the finite assets of a particular trust would be quickly eroded and the whole trust forced into dissolution for non-viability, that is, insolvency. In such a situation there is no guaranteed recourse to the government or anyone else. Negligence is not a risk that hospitals are permitted to insure against.

It may be that as the NHS patient is not a contracting party to the NHS trust or indeed GP fundholder, the chain of liability *vis-à-vis* patient and health authority remains unchanged and whatever claims would have lain against the health authority before the trust still exist. The position with regard to private patients, who are purchasers, might be more uncertain. It is perhaps only time that will decide and, unfortunately, a test case that will rationalise the position.

Generally speaking the intention of the NHS and Community Care Act 1990 is to pass control and responsibility to the management of NHS trusts and GP fundholders and for a greater degree of autonomy to exist for the individual unit divorced in the main from centralised control.

From training to education: a changed emphasis

In the educational sector of the health field, change has not been manifested in so tidy and absolute a way as in the provision of care. Nevertheless change has been far-reaching and in many ways has presented similar challenges to those administering health professional schooling.

Project 2000 must be hailed as an important focus for the change towards education away from on the job training in the schooling of nurses.

> The new Project 2000 curriculum will not only enhance the nursing profession's existing qualities, but also provide the opportunity to use more diverse forms of relevant knowledge.
>
> (Henry *et al.*, 1992, p92)

In the bid for independent professional status of nursing there is a renewed emphasis on caring rather than the previous focus which saw nurses as being merely supportive of the curing role of doctors. There is some evidence, though, of opposing views at play. The new style NHS, with its managerial emphasis on computerisation and hence standardisation, would seem to work against the move within nursing and, more particularly and arguably more successfully, within midwifery for professional autonomy amongst the caring professions. The new style education is working towards nurses and midwives with responsibility for the care of patients. Doctors in such a changed environment would have responsibility for the cure but not so much the care of patients. The arguments are more straightforward in the case of midwifery as, in the main, pregnant women are healthy. Doctors wanting to cure have a role only in the minority of abnormal pregnancies. Nurses are, of course, involved mostly with the care of unwell patients. The division of responsibility for care is thus more difficult to define. The process being carried out by hospital management would seem to be, however, towards identifying tasks previously carried out by nurses that need not be carried out by qualified staff. The result of this, far from enhancing the status of nurses as an independent profession, will be further to reduce the status of the former 'handmaidens'. Nurses must take on the struggle if true professionalism is to be acquired and/or retained by them.

If it is true to say that the government reforms are morally justified by a belief in patients, or clients as they are increasingly called, being asked to accept greater autonomy and responsibility for their own health care, then health professionals as the traditional providers of care must inherit this newly enhanced throne, jewelled by the government's economic priorities. They must be seen as experts and advisors to the public in matters of health care, occupying centre stage as carers but also as educators in preventive medicine. Only by these means do the ambitions and aims of health professionals coincide with those of government. In this way, by developing their role in prevention and care health professionals will carve out for themselves a distinct role different from that of doctors, whose continued emphasis ought properly to be on cure, complementary rather than subordinate and wholly deserving of professional status. Likewise the cultural priority in health will be at least equally on prevention and care, rather than on the over-wielding and expensive indulgence of science as was formerly the case, fostered in an atmosphere of doctor elitism.

The role of the new manager

As has been seen the legal position under the trusts casts the NHS manager in the role of service provider. Concentration is on performing the terms of the NHS contract operating between the trust and the relevant health authority. That relationship is thus only remotely governed by statutory obligation to provide care for the community, responsibility for which remains with the purchaser. The psychological change in the mind of the manager shifts from people to the provision of contracted units of care. The temptation to think in terms of 'x' number of operations rather than 'x' number of patients suffering from or in need of whatever is almost irresistible. The government who would promote autonomy, a philosophical principle associated with that of respect for persons, is here seen engineering a relationship whereby humans are measured according to object needs and as commodities of greater or lesser profitability.

If this temptation to regard persons is to be avoided it will surely be necessary for the NHS trust managers to have in place a clear ethical framework to which all personnel will have access and can use it as a basis for making decisions with regard to resources and standards of patient care. Ruth Chadwick states:

> It might be argued that in the specific context of priority setting in the health service the concept to turn to is efficiency rather than justice. It seems clear, however, that while efficiency is desirable it is also important to have a method of priority setting that is fair.
>
> (Chadwick, 1993, p85)

Organisational change, if not implemented by reference to ethical guidelines that have been accepted by all the individuals operating within an institution, can have a serious effect on the psychological contract operating in parallel with the legal contracts of employment (EVA Report, 1992). In the case of the NHS trusts it is not unlikely that the staff were formerly employed by the NHS as government employees. As has been stated the legislation pursuant to which the NHS trusts are set up insist that management shall have freedom to negotiate (with employees but not with trade unions or government) whatever terms of employment it thinks appropriate. The legal employment relationship between employees and NHS trusts will be different but it cannot be assumed that the terms of the psychological contract will be construed by employees to have changed. For example, where a new legal contract incorporates targets as part of the means of assessment of performance there will be a consequential change in the terms of the psychological contract. The ethos of employment will become more competitive and more individualistic. If that variation is not to lead to a destructive element undermining the employee's ability to work as part of a team, thereby decreasing the chance of increased efficiency rather than increasing it, employees will almost certainly need extensive retraining in the priorities and manifestations of the new ethos. Otherwise it is likely that personal insecurity and uncertainty, with regard to career expectations, will increase and impair the employee's ability to perform. If it is true that, under the terms of the new legal contract, the employment is more insecure than it was under the previous government terms, then management must be up front about that in encouraging employees to learn 'the rules' of the increasingly commercial environment. If old patterns of behaviour are no longer acceptable or sufficient that must surely be made clear. Managers themselves face similar changes in their own psychological contract. It can be argued that it is only against a background of sound ethical principles of fairness and respect that they will not fall into panic traps, whereby their decisions will be motivated entirely by survival concentrating on short-term goals disregarding the methods used or longer term consequences. For example, if there is an undue preoccupation with the 'numbers' game there will be a temptation to divert resources to quick, non-essential, possibly high profile, operations rather than on more time consuming essential operations.

The new managers will enter into contracts with the purchasers. Those contracts impose legal obligations on the providers to supply the commissioned services. It is important that the terms of the NHS contracts are compatible with the ethical principles adopted by the NHS trust. If this is not the case the priorities of managers to perform their legal obligations will constantly be at odds with the ethos and priorities of the doctors and health professionals involved in the provision of care. Clearly incompatible legal obligations will make it impossible for managers 'to practise what they preach'. The consequential tensions and stresses resulting from any incompatibility will doubtless impair the psychological contract in operation and it is likely that, sooner or later, disaster will be the outcome.

This illustrates, it is hoped, that it is essential that NHS trusts put in place a clear ethical framework at the earliest possible moment. To do so must surely provide the best recipe for success.

Similar challenges confront educational managers. Schools providing education have been attached to higher education institutions rather than the traditional location of training within the NHS. Incumbent upon them is the task of integrating the school into the culture of the university and also finding means whereby the old training orientation can be transformed into one where the aim is to educate professionals. It is perhaps appropriate here to talk about the function and role of codes of practice most often associated with the conduct of professionals.

The role of codes of practice

The Ormrod Committee in their report on Legal Education, 1971, stated:

> A profession involves a particular kind of relationship with clients, or patients, arising from the complexity of the subject matter which deprives the client of the ability to make informed judgements for himself and so renders him to a large extent dependent upon the

professional man. A self-imposed code of professional ethics is intended to correct the imbalance in the relationship between the professional man and his client and resolve the inevitable conflicts between the interests of the client and the professional man or of the community at large.

(The Law Society, 1974, p1)

Some would argue that our view of codes and professionals is rather different now. There has been, in recent years, an increasing emphasis on patient and client autonomy particularly with regard to informed consent. It can be argued that this has changed the power ratio operating between client and professional whereby the professional has less power and therefore less responsibility. Informed consent, whilst able to increase the patient's responsibility for what happens to him/her, at its worst can be used to relieve the professional of liability for what happens. This could be construed as converting the professional into a technician who is commissioned to provide a service but not to give advice.

When appraising the role of a code of practice it will first be necessary to have a clear understanding of the relationship between professional and client which the code is intended to govern. That there is debate about the role will presumably form part of the education programme of professionals, particularly that of health professionals, where the acknowledgement of them as professionals is in its infancy and indeed not without debate itself. Whether or not they are professionals is perhaps key to the change in emphasis from training to education.

The effect on the code of the analysis of the relationship will be one of degree rather than substance. One important aspect of a code is that it provides a guide as to the sort of behaviour the client may expect from a professional. Unfortunately it is not always the case that a code is available for the client to inspect. Ironically, too often, professionals themselves are ill-acquainted with the detailed content of a code. One exception to this is the code of the UKCC, which governs the conduct of nurses, midwives and district nurses. This code is commonly displayed in hospitals and other relevant places of work.

The unfamiliarity of professionals with their code, of course, implies that it is a code that has been imposed from the top rather than derived from the grass roots. It is argued in the EVA Report that a code will not be an effective tool for moral guidance unless those upon whom it is binding have had an effective opportunity to embrace its provisions (if not to devise them) and internalise the ethical principles embodied in them. It should also, the EVA Report argues, encompass shared values. Only in this way is a code able to give guidelines for human behaviour.

The role of Charters should be mentioned as they are becoming more and more prolific in both government and, particularly, private institutions. It can be argued that they can affect the power distribution between professional and client. They can also be viewed as instruments whereby the priorities of care imposed by managers are exposed to distortion. This idea is developed in Pritchard (1993).

Codes can be rewritten – a threatened outcome of changed priorities

The article in the *Observer* on Sunday 7th November 1993, about proposals to be put to the Ethics (sic) Committee of the British Medical Association, that patients who smoke or overeat will not be treated by doctors working in the NHS because such treatment is not 'cost-effective', cannot fail to send shivers down the spine of any right-thinking person. Hitler graced his policies of ethnic cleansing with some ideology, albeit fatally flawed: these doctors deny taking any moral stance and justify their proposals for 'cleansing' merely on grounds of economy.

The Ethics Committee of the BMA is being used to give credibility to a scheme which fundamentally changes the rationale of a doctor's role and of the NHS. Never have the tax payers who have paid for, and who continue to pay for the NHS, been consulted nor have they given any mandate to make these changes. No tax payer can escape some degree of responsibility for the state of her/his own health. Some philosophies, for example macrobiotics, ascribe responsibility for 'accidental' damage or injury to the body to an imbalance in a person's energy whereby the injury is 'brought' in order to correct the imbalance. Responsibility for one's own energy state rests with no-one but oneself. Consequently anyone involved in a car crash, be they driver, passenger or pedestrian, could be held responsible for the injury they sustain and found ineligible for treatment under the NHS if the proposals being put to the BMA are taken to their logical conclusions.

The doctors say they are not making moral judgements by prioritising patients according to their culpability but are prioritising according to the cost of treatment and if the patients' behaviour has resulted in poorer health, then the cost of treating them cannot be justified because their chances of obtaining long-term benefit are statistically reduced. Apparently one London surgery is not taking on any more mentally handicapped people. Clearly those patients cannot be blamed for their own mental retardation, if one follows accepted Western principles of causality: accordingly reference to culpability is not relevant. Nor can it be assumed that mentally handicapped patients are more expensive to treat than others or that they are less 'healthy'. What argument is this London doctor using? It must be assumed that this doctor, in imposing this embargo, regards such people as less worthy, less valuable human beings. Who is he to make such a judgement? How soon will other categories of 'less valuable human beings' be identified? Prostitutes, homosexuals, drug users . . . black prostitutes, black homosexuals, black drug users . . . black people. Historical English prejudice regards the Welsh as being dishonest and the Irish as being troublesome; are they 'less valuable'? Where will such policies end? There is no answer to that question. The only safe action is to prevent them from beginning.

The National Health Service was set up to provide health care for everybody, 'at no cost at the point of delivery', an expression the government is fond of using in its literature about the NHS trusts. Already, without detailed consultation with the electorate, NHS trusts have fundamentally changed the structure of the health service. The programme on BBC2 on 5th November 1993 called *Public Eye: The Health Business – A Question of Trust*, concerning the NHS trust run by Wellhouse in Edgware and Barnet, illustrates the dangers implicit in a structure where no-one is responsible. The government purchasers, namely the local health authority, escape liability by blaming the NHS trust management. The NHS management escape liability because, as a matter of law, they have no personal liability for the actions of the trust. The structure of the NHS trust allows the government to distance itself.

If the proposals discussed in the *Observer* article are accepted by the BMA Ethics Committee and are put into practice by doctors working in the NHS, NHS trust hospitals and/or NHS doctors' practices and/or GP fundholder practices, the government will not accept responsibility for the outrageously diminished health service available to untold, and as yet unidentified, members of the community. They will hide behind the 'managerial freedom' which was so generously given to trusts and GP fundholders by the legislation creating them.

In this example one role of codes is illustrated. They can be changed by their members. They can be used to govern conduct or they can be used to provide ethical guidelines. There is a great deal of diversity in the titles of codes whereby *conduct, practice* and *ethics* are used inconsistently. Harris sets out a useful guide as to how the various codes are used most helpfully.

> *Codes of Ethics:* 'In general, these consist of a fairly short set of broad ethical principles.' They contain statements stating what shall and shall not be done by each member.

> *Codes of Conduct:* These are generally far more detailed than Codes of Ethics. A broad ethical duty will be expanded to accommodate specific circumstances arising in practice.

> *Codes of Practice:* These will generally set out details of expected standards of behaviour or refer to the quality of work to be carried out by the profession. Interestingly such Codes are often directed at

the client base of the particular profession rather than used as a guide for members of the profession themselves.

(Harris, 1989, p5)

In the example above, the BMA are proposing alterations to a code of ethics. It can be argued that they are made more appropriately to a code of conduct. Conduct does not have to be moral whereas ethics clearly does. The assertion that doctors have an ethical duty to save money, which is stated in the article, is not true. They may have an ethical duty to use money fairly, but economy is not an ethical principle in itself. The judgemental way suggested for the means whereby economies will be made cannot be ascribed to ethics as it manifestly goes against the principles of liberty, autonomy and equal opportunity, not to mention respect for persons.

Conclusion

The reasons behind the 'reforms' in the NHS are obscured by party politics to a large degree. As the recession bites deeper that obscurity becomes more bitter. The purposes of this chapter must somehow be served without reference to political struggle. The origins of the 'reforms' are reputed to be found in the inefficient management structures which led to the appointment, first, of non-clinical managers and then to the formation of trusts and self-financing doctors' practices. It is argued by Loveridge and Starkey (1992) that the managerial crisis took place in inverse proportion to the medical success and advances in patient care.

> Moreover, the apparent lack of ability to discover administrative solutions for its multiplying problems has increasingly contrasted with the speed of innovation in the diagnosis and treatment of physical diseases within the NHS . . . The providers would obviously wish to retain the creativity and inventiveness of medical care-providers whilst structuring these activities in a manner that will allow for the greater standardisation and monitoring of performance.

(p2)

It is the balance between economic requirement and professional autonomy and integrity that is the subject of this discussion. The new-look NHS demands professionals with a revised outlook. The Government has legislated for educational changes which are designed to produce new thinking professionals. The dilemma for professionals is of course, whether or not high standards of care can be delivered within the demands of increased standardisation and an atmosphere of profit management.

Between professional care providers there are possible tensions as well as between management and health workers. Nurses, midwives and paramedics have traditionally been completely subservient to the wishes of doctors; arguably so has management. The historical position of the Royal Colleges and the British Medical Association is revealing:

> . . . at the same time the emphasis placed on the defence of the individual autonomy of their [Royal Colleges and NHS] members has tended towards encouraging a curative approach to health care management in which the doctor has retained his or her personal scope for judgement rather than a preventative or community-based perspective. This is a perspective which the new contracts offered to the profession by the Department of Health evidently seeks to redress.
>
> (Loveridge and Starkey, 1992, p8)

Thus it could be argued that with a greater emphasis on preventative care, there could be a levelling of the relative status of doctors and other health professionals within the NHS. The latter group has expertise in care rather than cure. If it can be shown that resources are better distributed in an NHS which has an increased emphasis on care, with impetus placed on education and prevention, then there may be not only greater autonomy given to health professionals but also greater autonomy given to the public at large. Through education the public are increasingly asked to take greater responsibility for their own individual health care. As this is a significant departure from the ethos of the NHS when it was set up in 1948 with its commitment to free health care for all, any such plan would have to be introduced slowly after proper preparation, possibly taking longer than a generation. The proposed change in emphasis is not undesirable *per se* but if introduced without due preparation will inevitably cause tremendous hardship whereby the tax payers, who have financed the NHS with certain expectations of care and cure, will be justifiably aggrieved. The danger in the present economic climate (and this is already being witnessed) is that the availability of facilities both for cure and hospital care are reduced before the community has been educated into looking after itself. For many people, it may be too late for prevention. Ethical principles cannot be found at this late stage to support the diminishment of cure when hitherto the culture has not supported care.

References

Chadwick, R. (1993) *Justice in Priority Setting*. In *Rationing in Action* BMJ Publishing Group, London.

Harris, N.G.E. (1989) *Professional Codes of Conduct in the United Kingdom*. Mansell Publishing, London, p.313.

HMSO (1979 and 1992) *Nurses, Midwives and Health Visitors Acts*.

HMSO (1990a) *NHS and Community Care Act*.

HMSO (1990b) *Working for Patients. NHS Trusts: A Working Guide*.

HMSO (1992) *The Patient's Charter*.

The Law Society (1974) *A Guide to the Professional Conduct of Solicitors*. The Law Society, London.

Loveridge, R. and Starkey, K. (eds) (1992) *Continuity and Crisis in the NHS*. Open University Press, Buckingham.

Pritchard, J. (1993) *Charters, Charters and More Charters!* Paper, International Conference on Professional and Business Ethics, University of Central Lancashire, October, 1993.

Editor's note to Chapter 3

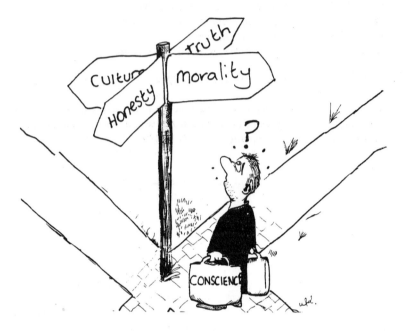

Chapters 1 and 2 have introduced both the theory and practical application of applied ethics, particularly in the professional setting; Chapter 3 will bring this first section on theory and practice to a close. Stylistically rather different from the rest of the book, that difference in itself exemplifies its own message; namely that language has an intrinsic ability to distort. Language will be the means whereby both theory and practice are communicated; the next chapter warns the reader of the inescapable subjectivity of the tool itself.

Ethics may itself be an ideal; this chapter argues that any communication in words will take imperfection further. The terms we use are always value laden. Care must be taken to minimise any 'hidden agendas'. The chapter is written by one of the members of the EVA and the discussion is set in the context of how language was used in the project and how we sought to avoid the pitfalls.

Whilst considering the arguments of the next chapter the reader is invited to consider how the language itself is used and note the effect that has. Whilst doing this the reader should imagine how ethical principles themselves and any rendering of them could be distorted and/or changed by different linguistic presentations.

3 Language and ethics

George Campbell

"I don't know what you mean by 'glory,'" Alice said. Humpty Dumpty smiled contemptuously. "Of course you don't – till I tell you. I meant 'there's a nice knock-down argument for you!'" "But 'glory' doesn't mean 'a nice knock-down argument'," Alice objected. "When I use a word," Humpty Dumpty said, in a rather scornful tone, "it means just what I choose it to mean – neither more nor less." "The question is," said Alice, "whether you can make words mean so many different things." "The question is," said Humpty Dumpty, "which is to be master – that's all."

(Carroll, 1984, p100)

Introduction

The hypothesis of this chapter is that language is so interrelated to the concepts it is used to manifest that it is virtually impossible to give an objective account of anything. The title 'Language and ethics' can itself have several meanings. The context is the world of work. This chapter will concentrate on how language is used and give examples to show how influential language is in effecting relationships as well as describing them. Acknowledging the difficulty, it will then attempt to find effective values in language. Finally it will look at how language was experienced during the EVA Project and how, in the collection and analysis of data, language was attempted to be used ethically.

Language and the world of work

In the microcosms of work and the home the same negotiations are going on. When the process fails in the domestic sphere we have family breakdown. This may result in divorce and the language of recrimination. It may show itself in the lack of control of children by parents and a lack of control within the children themselves. The parents will resort to the language of authoritarianism, the children to the language of rebellion. Language judges behaviour: it may control by threats of violence or be the empty rhetoric of threat: it could be the language of reconciliation and persuasion. The separation of behaviour and language can be argued as being artificial. For most people language is a form of behaviour that expresses emotions about, and evaluations of, situations. (Emotions in themselves are one mode of evaluation.) This is the realm of 'private' morality.

In the world of work the debates are not only about the duties and the responsibilities for which wages or salary is paid but also about the way in which those duties and responsibilities are created, enacted and ended. When this fails we are often in the emotionally fraught world of strikes, lock-outs, arbitration and industrial tribunals. This is the realm of professional ethics.

Professional ethics deals with those areas of social behaviour within the world of work which are not enshrined in law. It deals with the social contract which is enacted between the managers and the managed. It is deeply dependent on the way each party, or individual, perceives their 'contractual' rights and, generally, the correlative duties. Operating outside any contractual situation are, too, the relationships which exist between employees and managers amongst themselves. The EVA Report refers to this extra-legal contract as the 'psychological contract'.

Aspects of the psychological contract are harassment (including sexual) and prejudice. Language clearly plays a focal part in how these are manifested. Ironically they are very often not taken seriously if they are taken no further than language. It can be argued though, that harassment, in whatever form , is the exercise of power, very often the abuse of power. A person harassing another may do so to enhance his or her own sense of power; sometimes there is an attempt to ignore the unethical aspects of the encounter. It is called 'teasing', referred to as 'only a joke'. Sometimes the 'blame' for the harassment is transferred to the victim, for example, using phrases like, 'Can't you take a joke?' commonly said with varying amounts of aggression. This notion of 'teasing' appears again used against the victim where, in some rape cases, the alleged 'teasing' of the rapist by the victim has been proffered by the rapist as a defence and, even more disempowering of the victim, is held as amounting to consent!

Aspects of language

Ethics deals with the abstract links between people. Its presence, or absence, plays an extremely important role in their relationships. The difficulty with language has already been pointed out. Clearly where language must present abstract concepts the problems multiply. The following subsections illustrate the part played by language in some of the concepts where ethics seeks to be heard. It will be noted that many of the examples refer to the family. It is perhaps in some notion of seeking to resist a rather popular executive delusion 'that morality is left at home when one goes to work' that makes this setting appropriate together with the rather holistic ethic that work is a wider circling of the family unit.

In these examples the reader is asked to become immersed in the language and then to stand back from the language and consider the use of some words compounded with other slightly different words used in similar situations, and to note also how the same word can be used to mean different things in different contexts. The reader is then asked to consider how changing language can actually change the nature of rights, particularly those associated with work and more especially those associated with the psychological contract.

Symbols

Language is a form of communication between people in order to bring about certain acts and to generate certain beliefs. This is not completely or solely a human facility. In many ways animals have the means to communicate with each other, mostly on an instinctive and evolved basis and strictly limited in range.

Some baboons for instance have different cries of warning which indicate generally whether danger is above, a bird of prey perhaps; below, creatures like snakes or ground predators; in the trees, or their locality. Such a series of cries may be learned and may or may not change. Certainly whether it is the nest of a bower bird or the cry of a baboon, the communication does not compare in complexity and purpose with human language. There is now a long history of research into the communication capacities of chimpanzees and it has been argued that their skills in this area have little to do with survival in terms of obtaining enough food and protecting themselves from a hostile environment; their signing and signalling skills in their natural habitat are used to enhance the collective commitment of the group to its members and of the members' commitment to the group. In other words, the 'language' of these near kin in the animal world is devoted not so much to survival as to social interaction. (Gardner *et al.*, 1989; Jones, 1993).

Without wishing to sound sentimental it would seem that the evolution of human language will never be known and can only be speculated on. Certainly at some stage the nearly human creatures who first used a sound or other symbol for something that was not to hand, took a giant step forward for mankind. Consider telling a friend about your holiday and look at all the symbols and signs you can bring to bear – language, postcards, photographs, mementoes, even trying to relive the experience by use of a videotape. You are trying to give someone a sense of the vividness of something that is now absent and is in the past. It can be argued that language is the main element in our individual memories and our national and cultural histories.

Indeterminacy and arbitrariness

When philosophers like Wilburn (1947) began the study of language
they found it to be arbitrary, dependant on social agreement, as well as
being part of the foundation of memory and judgement. This sense of
the instability and arbitrariness of language became very important for
philosophers and the developing sciences.

Language was thought to be arbitrary because it derived from
agreed social conventions and indeterminate because meaning resided
in the agreement of the memories of all the language users. There was
a great longing to 'know' the real world, not as described by the senses
or by language but in itself. Despite considerable efforts on the part of
many philosophers it has proved impossible, simply on language
grounds, to justify or prove anything beyond the social and 'natural'
life of man and woman in the world as it is described, or inscribed, by
our sign systems, which are not restricted to words. For some, relying
on a religious faith can take many people beyond this multicentred
relativistic universe but many are left viewing the world through the
'spectacles' of language, in both senses of that word.

What Saussure did at the beginning of the century was to suggest
the inseparability of the idea from the sound of the spoken word. He
collapsed together the notion of an idea of a thing and the sound of it
when spoken. So that idea/word becomes a 'sign'. This sign was then
considered to be defined not so much by its reference to a thing as by its
difference from other similar sounds. An understanding of this can be
obtained by changing one letter of a word in sequence to obtain its
opposite. Love – hate. Love, lave, (obsolescent words allowed!), late,
hate. This shows that **love** is defined as the opposite of hate in dictionary
terms, but in terms of sound it is defined by the sound field around it;
defined by how it differs from words like live, leave, loaves, laugh,
glove, etc. as well as by 'common sense' usage.

What this emphasises is the social nature of language. From Socrates
and Plato onwards the meaning of language as used by society to define
'good' behaviour and its opposite has been a central question in the
discussions of philosophy.

Women as an example of gender

Recently the University of Central Lancashire held a conference on
the subject of consensual sexual relations between university staff and
students. Issues of privacy and possible abuse of knowledge or power
were significant in the discussions.

An extension of such power, perhaps, is the notion of political
correctness; for example, how language is used in relation to the
equality of women. The 'politically correct' seek to reduce those
elements in the language that debase and 'infantalise' women. In this

way they try to tackle the ethical problems of value directly. Currently when women refer to themselves or are referred to by others as 'girls' they can be admonished because the word 'infantilises' them. This seems to mistake the way language works and to create questions of rights. It should be asked firstly, who has the right to determine 'disparity of language' in a democratic country and by what authority?

It is possible to define words as unacceptable and enshrine that, in principle, within law. In libel and slander, for example, and in terms of using racist language, there are legal constraints, but this normally happens after a society has been persuaded that the use of certain words is wrong. Until then persuasion and example are the only sensible ways forward.

Secondly, people use language as social bonding – not as a set of dictionary meanings. If women want to strengthen their social network by using the diminutive of woman, viz. 'girl' or 'girls', they are using language as it develops their social life. By all means debate the issue but to instruct or even to exercise 'moral pressure,' it can be argued, is to destroy the basis of the argument, for such activities debase and 'infantalise' the recipient more than the use of the word itself. Alternatively, if the argument of this chapter has any merit, namely that language indeed is powerful enough to effect change, then a man calling grown women 'girls' has the effect of making them into children and, as such, arguably gives them the same amount of power in society as children rather than the greater share usually afforded to adults and the context matters.

The list of words that disparage women directly, in terms of their meaning, such as 'tart', 'bimbo', 'scrubber' and the like, is much longer than the list of words that really disparage men. It is this area of language that should be addressed. The words condemn individual women for behaving in ways that the users of such language often find praiseworthy when the behaving is done by men. The language itself bears witness to the double standards in operation.

Ownership

One of the more interesting perceptions is the view of 'ownership.' There has been an ideological divide in Britain for many years about public and private ownership. It is assumed, for example, that there is greater freedom to act within the 'market' for private companies. All these perceptions are based on the concept of the type of ownership of a company. Yet the word itself is not as simple as at first appears and has within it implications of rights and limitations. The language of ownership gives disposable rights but also falsifies relationships.

The owner of a Chippendale chair has the right as 'owner' to burn it on a cold night to keep warm; the owner of a painting by an internationally renowned artist, whilst quite free to burn the painting, may be restricted if there is an attempt to remove the painting from the country and sell it abroad.

It has in the past been considered acceptable to 'own' slaves. In some cases the law considers children to 'belong' to their parents. A child is perhaps not 'owned' by the parent but is in some sense the parent's. If the parent fails to do his or her parental duty, the child will be put into the 'care' of the state. Who owns the child then? Implicit in the situation is the idea of custody; children are taken into custody. Custodianship is an accountable role. Who gives the 'state' rights over a child; rights which can take precedence in certain circumstances over those of the parents? Collectively the members of this society have agreed that the 'authorities' have rights to curb and support a parent's behaviour. In some states the authority is expressed in language that roots the power in the decisions of the people, for example in Abraham Lincoln's famous phrase, 'Government of the people, by the people, for the people'. Does this give the state rights over an individual, even though that individual may not have consented to that authority? Does the state 'own' the people?

Power

It has been shown that the exercise of 'ownership' or 'custodianship' is the exercise of 'authority'. Most authority is given or created in order to manage events and people. Management is the exercise of power. Shareholders, for example, in large companies delegate their power to paid managers, whose function it is to exercise power in the 'market' for the benefit of their employers. The implementation of the simplest office or business procedure involves instructions to carry out certain actions, to perform in certain ways. The way these instructions and transactions are carried out is part of the realm of professional and business ethics.

Government is also the exercise of power, with or without the consent of a majority of the population governed. When the central authority breaks down there can be civil strife, as in Bosnia, for example. Taxation and the implementation of policy at home and abroad are, in democratic countries, exercised with the will of an elected government. This should also be part of the realm of professional ethics.

These are not the only centres of power in any community. To think that institutions, for example a university or other large employer, operating within the state do not exercise power within their bureaucracies is a misperception. It can be argued that wherever power is exercised is the concern of ethics. Professional ethics leaves aside power bases like the family and concentrates on the public domain. Within this domain there are in operation a great proliferation of codes of behaviour, both formal and informal. It is clear that if the implications of the power of language are that language can shape 'interiority' or the inner life of a 'subject' or person and are even partially true, then the way we look at those who transgress these codes of behaviour must include an understanding of the way that the transgressor has developed his or her perceptions of an ethical or moral world.

Where an individual or group is engaged in the exercise of power, either as owner or custodian, either privately or publicly, the medium of the exercise of power is language.

Looking for values

Given the social creation of the way the individual is developed and the way that the individual affects the social process, can we ever be certain of creating sustainable ethical values? In a multicultural world, is it possible to produce a set of understandings that can be honoured universally? The notion of ethnicity, as this carries with it differences of race, is not discussed here because it is a larger issue than can be dealt with in this chapter and biologically speaking, there is really very little difference between human societies in terms that make the discussion of the gene pool relevant. The issue of racist language is one the writer is reluctant to comment upon, belonging as I do to the powerful so-called 'White Anglo-Saxon Protestant' community which seems to have power, any careless expression is open to misreading and may cause more opacity than clarity. Suffice it to say at this point that the language contains many more expressions that use black negatively than use white negatively and to be balanced *he* wants neither to be a 'blackguard' nor a 'whited sepulchre'.

There is a greater biological difference between women and men than between the so-called races, yet the shadowing (in physiological terms) between the sexes makes the vast majority of differences we perceive socially generated rather than biologically given. Women's 'rights' are determined by the amount of power they can exert in the whole community. Belonging to any group which has rights in terms of the larger society means that often control is exerted by that larger group. In many communities children are not fully 'human' until certain rituals have taken place. They are in a 'liminal' state (Growler, 1972). During illness an individual's 'autonomy' can be lost by becoming a 'patient'. It is significant that this is not the way the individual perceives him or herself, but the way the caring group gives identity to that person.

It is clear that in such an area the individual choice is not an act of private morality. The range of expertise involved is great, and social rather than private decisions have to be made. For example, should the state allow a service to develop privately or be publicly funded? Given the ability to perform certain acts to generate a fetus in technical rather than 'natural' ways, would the morality governing their development be based on principles of defining the human being?

If the person(s) make moral or ethical decisions on grounds other than that of materialism, they are in the difficulty of determining the authority of the decision. The authority may come from a sacred text, whatever the religion, and Marxism is included in this on the grounds that 'history' is often seen as somehow transcendental in that thinking. Other structures may be offered as to the basis of morality within the human sphere by believers in religion. These, like all beliefs, will be moulded by the cultural atmosphere in which the believers grow up. No matter how the arguments are put together, the definition of a 'person' in such a community transcends the biological functioning of the human entity. Such groups may make the decision that only 'natural' means may be used. For such people genetic moulding may be untenable but artificial insemination acceptable, though fertilisation outside the womb may present difficulties (Nuttall, 1993).

Even if it is conceded that persons have individual being and are id-entities, it must also be acknowledged that they are the products of intense acculturation with the semiotic system creating our discriminations and perceptions. Values are also made within the semiotic system. Is it acceptable that the apparent stability brought by power and authority and ownership should determine our lives (Berlin, 1993), or should persons seek to affirm the value of sharing and democracy, custodianship and debate, thereby affirming the desire for the autonomy that Kant so clearly defines as a value in his essay, 'what is enlightenment'? (Kant, 1984).

Do persons really believe in these words of self-hood and autonomy in the quotidian reality of the trivial round and the common task?

The EVA Project

When approaching the study and analysis of the implicit ethical values of a group it cannot be assumed that there are any given authorities. Religious and cultural norms can be used descriptively but should not be used prescriptively. In a multicultural society there may well be conflicting cultural norms or religious injunctions. When the Ethics and Values Audit was set up at the University of Central Lancashire it was clear to the team that no easy answer was to be found in terms of what were and what were not acceptable behaviours, nor was it clear as to how an act or behaviour pattern could be analysed in ethical terms. The university mission statement and other codes of practice in terms of research, harassment and other procedures laid out general guidelines. However, interpretation could be ambiguous and it was not clear that the guidelines and codes were practised in effect.

The first process was to create a questionnaire which would give some understanding of whether or not there existed any values that were shared by the university community, how its members viewed their working environment and the social situation at work, and how the community 'distributed' its values in the everyday life world contained in its functioning.

Lists of topics were developed which related to some purported values which were thought to be relevant; these were refined and a process of questioning developed from them. It was immediately recognised that there was a major problem in trying to generate questions which did not carry within them a prejudgement or an implied answer. It is this problem which is central to this chapter, because language is itself a discriminatory tool used by people in very wide-ranging and subtle ways.

The shared values of a community are not readily accessible. They are embodied in the way documents are written, the way people respond to communications and to each other, both formally and informally. The values are a set of perceptions which embody the polarities of cynicism and uncritical acceptance. They are not necessarily best shown in statements of intent, nor in the most negative comments. Any group who wishes to examine its shared assumptions must look carefully at its aims and goals, and above all the language in which it expresses them.

During the course of the audit, the team set out to determine the shared values in our community, which we did by processes which ranged from the use of statistical data to personal case study material. To do so the team had to try to use language in a non-authoritarian way and in a way that did not pre-empt the answers.

The team could not delineate a set of values and see how they were implemented nor could it, in a multiethnic community, choose one set of perceptions rather than another.

The language of data collection

In devising a questionnaire the audit team sought to create as neutral a set of statements as was possible. These statements were related to working practices, working relationships and resources and income generation. As the questionnaire developed it became clear that the way forward at that time was to generate a situational analysis in terms of satisfaction with the variety of situations community members found themselves in. To some this appeared to be a morale questionnaire and to some extent this was true. The team devised a set of criteria in terms of *culture* (referring to the whole institution), *management* (referring to all the managerial processes), *knowledge* (all aspects of information), *autonomy* (relating to respect for persons), *self-affirmation* (the rights of individuals to be affirmed as persons irrespective of role), *images of other people* (dealing with our individual perception of others), and *values* (the importance we place on the choices we make in terms of the above.) These terms are more fully defined in the *EVA Report*, pp.42–3. These criteria were carefully defined after much discussion and provided the basis upon which the implicit values were described.

The use of a value grid, based upon Kelly (1955), specifically addressed the values held by individuals. The results of this process supported those of the questionnaire. This is not the place to analyse the findings, but to concentrate on the language we used to develop the team's understandings. Unlike the commonsense perception that words have an opposite, the team found it could only define what it considered a positive value, as some values could be seen as a balance between opposites. For example, being assertive was seen as a positive value between being unassertive and aggressive, i.e. being able to defend one's position without anger.

This enabled the team to group responses. The confidential data drawn from the interviews and problem cases were analysed by the group, who were able, on the basis of the definitions built up by the questionnaire and the values grid, to identify both the apprehensions and aspirations of those involved in the structured interviews and 'hotline' case studies.

One of the recommendations of the Report was that communication should be open. Openness of communications and information flow is crucial to a healthy community, large or small. Control of information is a form of power, which makes the mission statement's commitment to openness a significant contribution to the health of the community.

The team was clear what the University community would like to see but the development of an ethically determined 'ethos' and 'culture' has to be addressed by the whole community (Wilcox and Ebbs, 1992).

The base line of ethical understanding that the report underlined at all levels was that:

the person should be respected
and that abuse of power and role should be condemned.

This cannot hope to be done unless we understand the pitfalls which can be created by the community itself if it neglects the language in which it attempts to embody its values.

Conclusion

It has been shown therefore that the way language is used changes the meaning it is able to give. Seemingly innocent phrases used every day in common parlance, when analysed, can be shown to be ripe, even festering, with prejudice and offence. The EVA Project tried its best to be sensitive and conscious in its use of language. In the actual conduct of the project, of course, many forms of communication were available other than the written word; the personal interview, for example, where body language can play a part. This chapter is confined, like the printed EVA Report, to the language of paper. It is hoped that language was used ethically. In addition, by drawing attention to the almost integral prejudices and non-ethics in language it is hoped that greater vigilance will be used by those who would not merely speak ethically but be ethical. Let there not be an overindulgence, though, in linguistic political correctness, lest that fool who rushed in to do good is dissuaded from trying again!

It can be seen from the argument, therefore, that a user of language must be careful about the language of morality and must be careful of the morality of language. The virtually intrinsic involvement of language and values makes it inevitable that each position implies the other.

It is as if our view of ourselves is internalised from the mirrors of the society around us. The mirror is looked into and ourselves defined and, if the mirrors are tainted, that colouring can be assumed either for better or for worse. The unfortunate thing is that each one of us is also a mirror to each other, offering a tainting of the surface or the opaqueness of 'respectability'. The language by which we and others are defined seems to be the surface of this mutual reflexivity. Perhaps all that can be done in the end is to try to make sure that one's personal bit of the surface is kept as reflective as possible.

> Morality regains its vigour when ordinary people have learnt afresh to decide for themselves what principles to teach their children. But there will be some changes, some of the principles of the rebels will have been adopted. That is how morality progresses – or retrogresses. The process is . . . reflected by the very subtle changes in the uses of value words.
>
> (Hare, 1964, pp73–74)

References

Berlin, I. (1993) *The Crooked Timber of Humanity, Chapters in the History of Ideas*. Vintage Books, Random House, New York.

Carroll, L. (1984 edn.) *Alice Through the Looking Glass*. Puffin Classics, Penguin Books, London.

Gardner, R.A., Gardner, B. and van Cantfort, T.E. (1989) *Teaching Sign Language to Chimpanzees*. University of New York Press, New York.

Growler, D. (1972) On the concept of being a person. In *Six Approaches to the Person*, R. Ruddock (ed.) Manchester University Press, Manchester.

Hare, R.M. (1964) *The Language of Morals*. Oxford University Press, Oxford.

Jones, J. (1993) *Chimp Talk*. BBC Horizon Publication, BBC, London.

Kant, E. (1984) 'What is Enlightenment?' In *German Aesthetic and Literary Criticism; Kant, Fichte, Schelling, Schopenhaur, Hegel*. Cambridge, D. Simpson (ed.) pp.29–34. Cambridge University Press, Cambridge.

Kelly, G. (1955) *The Psychology of Personal Constructs*. Norton, New York.

Locke, J. (1964 edn.) Book III, Of Words. p.200f.) *An Essay Concerning Human Understanding. 1690*. Everyman.

Nuttall, J. (1993) *Moral Questions, An Introduction to Ethics*. Polity Press & Blackwell, Cambridge.

Saussure, F. (1992) A general course on linguistics. In *A Critical and Cultural Reader*, A. Easthope and K. McGowan (eds.) Open University Press, Buckingham.

Wilburn, R. (1947) Book III, of Words – John Locke. *An Essay Concerning Human Understanding*, pp.201–246. J.M. Dent & Sons Ltd, London.

Wilcox, J.R. and Ebbs, S.L. (1992) *The Leadership Compass. Values and Ethics in Higher Education*. George Washington University, Washington, DC.

Section Two
Managing change

Editor's note to Section Two

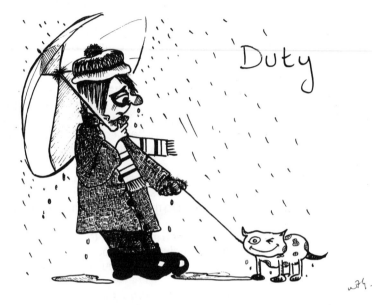

The theory and practice of professional ethics has been discussed in Section One with an example of organisational change being shown in Chapter 2; this section will concentrate on how organisational change could, perhaps should, be managed. The EVA Project is cited as an example of a very practical way change can be tackled. It argues strongly in favour of grass root consultation to avoid the danger of a workforce enveloped by structural change becoming disillusioned and alienated from the developments being instigated by management. To some degree the recommendations of the EVA which emerge from this section are foreshadowed by the theoretical position discussed in Chapter 1 and the effect of change in the Health Service particularly in relation to employment contracts and the parallel psychological contract referred to in Chapter 2. Likewise they are followed through in the aspirational examples of how they might apply in practice contained in Section Three.

   Chapter 4 outlines with practical emphasis what the EVA is about and what it does. It explains how effective an ethics and values audit can be when used as an ethical management tool. The reader is referred to Appendix 2 which sets out a full summary of the EVA, with the exception of the actual methods used, which are dealt with in

Appendix 1. There is reference to a public perception that both health and educational organisation are caring communities. It takes up the central question of the EVA, namely 'Do [they] practise what [they] preach?'. The chapter carries on discussion of codes begun in Section One, adding charters and mission statements to the frame.

Chapter 5 takes up the managerial theme in both higher education and the health service but this time specifically from a management perspective. It illustrates how the problems caused by change in complex organisational structures can be assessed and evaluated through the audit process. It emphasises an EVA as a means whereby one of the major problems, namely a lack of shared values, can be minimised, the absence of which can be very obstructive to the successful introduction of change. It shows how an EVA can be an important means of achieving a sincerely held corporate culture. It contrasts the modern view of corporate identity to atomistic individualism.

A social scientist's perspective of organisational change is provided by Chapter 6 whilst Chapter 7 views the EVA through the eyes of a teacher of health professionals, also the subject of change as was referred to in Chapter 2.

Chapter 6 concentrates on the search in the EVA to identify values shared by the people working in the university. It goes on to relate the findings to education in general with its new focus on principles of openness, diversity and choice.

Chapter 7 draws neatly together the two examples of organisational change featured in this book through the position of the people

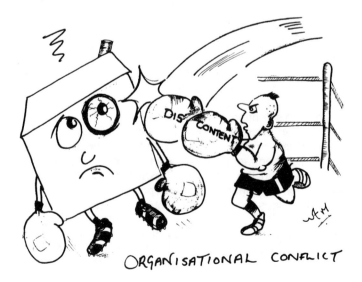

ORGANISATIONAL CONFLICT

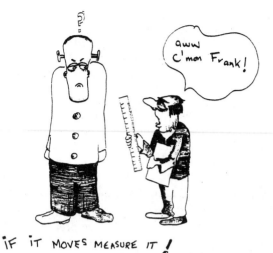

IF IT MOVES MEASURE IT !

who must somehow cope with both changes, namely those involved in educating the new health professional. Some mention of this role was made in Chapter 2 and again is implicit in Chapter 10 but here is expanded and related specifically to the EVA. It carries on the emphasis on shared values found in the previous chapters in this section.

This whole section provides real situations where the theory behind the EVA is challenged with practical implementation.

4 An introduction to the ethics and values audit (EVA)

Christine Henry and Janine Drew

Practising what we preach

This chapter focuses upon the development of an ethical management tool (an ethics and values audit) that attempts to facilitate improvement in professional practice within the organisation, giving direction for examining whether we practise what we preach.

Within current NHS and higher education organisational change, whilst the value of care is 'preached' in one establishment, another 'competition' may be practised (Henry *et al.*, 1992). In becoming a professional there is an implicit duty to practise within a moral frame of reference. Members of the organisation's community, including leaders of that organisation, are subjected to the structure and the processes from within and to the pressure and demands from without. Furthermore, external ideological, political and economic factors impose their own influences on personal, professional and organisational integrity. From a professional perspective, there is personal and collective accountability for maintaining and establishing the standards of practice. There ought to be shared professional and organisational values but how are we able to identify these?

According to Wilcox and Ebbs (1992) the word 'profession' has an historical origin within a religious community. This directly relates to being a member of a particular community and to the making of a commitment of a particular kind. Religious and educational communities and health professions follow rules of caring. Furthermore, the general public and the professionals themselves may generally perceive the NHS hospital and educational institutions as caring communities.

In chapter 1, it was seen that central to ethical practice and the idea of a caring community is an understanding of important moral principles and values. It is essential for both moral integrity and creditability for assessing good practice that shared principles and values are implicit within the professional codes and the organisation's mission statement, if there is a serious attempt to practise what we preach.

Charters, mission statements and codes

Professional standards and codes are usually perceived as guidelines to generally accepted norms. According to Bellah *et al.*, (1985) charters and codes are often necessary when a culture is undergoing change and where a lack of consensus of values may become evident.

Charters are statements that involve a summary of good practice and the identification of standards. A charter will reach a wider audience and is broadly interprofessional in essence. The Patient's Charter (DoH, 1991) is a guide identifying standards aimed to improve and modernise the delivery of health care. A charter will reaffirm fundamental principles and values. However, difficulties arise both in their construction and implementation, if they are imposed upon an organisation from 'top down' without a sense of ownership by the members of that organisation's community. Identifying standards and ways to improve those standards ought to be encouraged through research based value audits that capture the values, principles and perceptions of all the stakeholders within and across NHS and educational organisations. The same process may be applied to mission statements.

Whilst mission statements are broad statements of intent they form the first phase in a process that attempts to enhance practising what we preach. However, the most obvious criticism arises where the mission statement is totally at odds with the behaviour of the specific members of the organisation.

Codes are specific to particular professional groups. Like charters, codes set guidelines for standards and must have identified principles that underpin practice. The nurses' Code of Professional Conduct as a guideline for good practice is still not widely known nor its purpose appreciated by individuals within the profession. According to Heywood Jones (1990), knowing the code gives personal advantage and benefit to the profession as a whole. It is the responsibility of every practitioner to conform to the code; those who violate it may find themselves the subject of peer investigation. This self-professional scrutiny is based upon the principle of respect for and protection of the public. Likewise the same may be applied to an organisation mission statement and any organisational code. A code extends the perimeters of a charter by giving directives to the professional and is concerned with professional regulation and the individual's professional conduct. Codes therefore must be continually evaluated and monitored and the guidelines explicitly stated so that directives may be taken to guide practice.

Mission statements, charters and codes may well form at least part of the process of practising what we preach. However, it seems highly relevant and perhaps essential to find ways in which existing charters, mission statements and codes can be evaluated, monitored or modified and credible processes in which new codes and charters can be developed. There is some requirement for identifying organisational values in order to develop realistic mission statements, charters or codes that will enhance good practice and in turn raise the ethical profile of the profession and the organisation. A major ethical concern lies with formulating a charter, a mission statement or a code that is not already owned by the members of the community. It may be perceived as imposed upon the members, arriving 'out of thin air'. The members either are unsure how it has been constructed or have not participated in its development. One of the problems that arises and causes conflict is that of mismatch between organisational and professional values. In some cases a sense of helplessness arises if the mission statement, charter or code is unrealistic and cannot be put into practice.

An ethical management tool: the Ethics and Values Audit (EVA)

Do we practise what we preach? It is from this question that the Ethics and Values Audit (EVA) evolved. The EVA is a management tool that facilitated an examination and identification of shared principles and values underpinning mission statements, charters and codes. Furthermore, it can be seen as the first stage in a process for managing change. Wilson (1993) remarks that:

> In years to come when many more organisations may be conducting ethical audits the EVA will be seen as the first serious attempt to quantify the profound effects ethics and values have on both organisational behaviour and performance

> (p103)

The NHS and the education sector are constantly facing change with the inevitable effect it has on the professional within the organisation. Apps (1993) remarks that although the EVA took place in an institute of higher education it has much to offer nursing and health care professional practice. The EVA may be applied to all professionals within the NHS including those managing the service. The EVA examines something fundamental to an organisation's stability, i.e. the facilitation of both staff and clients' awareness of their own moral lives and those of the organisation's culture. Wilcox and Ebbs (1992) state that morality not only concerns individual and social welfare but is very much a part of the institutional landscape. Given the vital role of NHS and education organisations within our society and the mission emanating from that role, it is crucial that special attention is given to the ways in which goals are achieved and obligations to society fulfilled. Implicit within the moral charter granted by society to the organisation is the enhancement of the common good, through its primary activity in the delivery of health care and education. An EVA is the beginning of an ongoing process of self-evaluation.

The EVA questions the notion of whether a highly moral corporate culture exists within any organisation and how any organisation is able to uphold and achieve its mission when it is faced with social, economic and political pressures. Furthermore, it addresses some of the problems that arise when market forces are imposed upon the public sector services. It is clearly identified that the impetus for the Ethics and Values Audit emerged from a recognition of 'the perception of a double standard, the impact of change and the sensitivity to values and moral life that characterise these times' (Henry *et al.*, 1992 p2).

Henry *et al.*, remark that the process of identifying and exploring values and principles involves research analysis and debate in discovering ways to enhance ethical practice within an organisation. Organisations attempt to enhance their professional standing by presenting a high ethical profile by adhering to their mission, charters and codes of practice. This is crucial both for the health care and education organisations and their professional members, particularly in times of change. What we do, in addition to what we say, provides the application of implementing values into practice.

The EVA was based upon four premises involving the identification of values underpinning an organisation's mission statement, how the values are shared and practised, the staff's and clients' perceptions of values and how the organisation would better fulfil its responsibilities to the society it serves. The objectives included producing a profile of shared values supported by ethical principles, an examination of organisational policy, recommending ways to enhance policy and practices and an understanding of ethical issues and ways to resolve the problem.

The project was research based and involved capturing the day-to-day concerns of the organisation. The main ethical principle is respect for and dignity of persons, as well as recognition of the needs of the organisation. The outcome of the EVA resulted in a three part comprehensive report.

Part One examines the purpose of the project, identifying the aims and presenting the results of the research based audit through ten themes highly relevant to the specific organisation. These themes identified issues regarding informal networks, mutual respect and trust, peer group integrity, honesty and openness, interpersonal relationships, organisational decision making processes, styles of management, management practice, use and abuse of power and the provision of resources. Whilst these themes are of specific value to the individual organisation, the development of a profile may be transferable to other organisations. Wilson (1993) remarks that the process of an ethics audit maps out how values are shared between goals and objectives of an organisation and codes and the individual's own values and beliefs. Not only is it important to identify the shared values but also those values that are not the same. Whilst the quality of the shared values, goals and activities are reflected in and through the working relationships within the organisation, the differently held values, if viewed as conflicting, will also be reflected through achieved goals of the organisation.

The EVA Report at the beginning of Part One states that if the organisation's attitude does not match how staff see themselves and their role, co-operation will eventually be withdrawn. Furthermore, if psychological needs are ignored and misunderstanding and poor communication ensue, endless conflicts arise. The EVA was in one sense a preventive strategy, in that examining the organisational culture, finding out both positive and negative aspects, it seemed realistic to develop an action plan or a list of recommendations that could address some of the issues of concern. A cluster of values derived from the interviews and a value grid identified principal values which the organisation could practise in order to encourage a more stable psychological contract with the members of the organisation. The values identified included openness, good communication, collaboration, responsibility, respect, awareness, being valued, trust, integrity, accountability and professionalism. One respondent stated: 'One qualitative aspect is that we have got ethics on the agenda and that to me is a positive aspect of the institution which has accepted its responsibilities' (Henry *et al.*, 1992, p9).

The analysis of the data allowed for a credible list of recommendations which included issues related to styles of leadership and management, ways of improving the organisational culture, a review of the mission statement and the development of an organisational code of practice which should be consistent with the mission statement, policy statements and the organisation's charter for management initiative. Further recommendations involved ways to improve communication, development of a learning community, ways to improve the environment and an ethics and values audit for students. The recommendations where open for debate and crossorganisational seminars were arranged, encouraging feedback from staff.

> The recommendations are not (nor could be) explicitly ethical or moral. They represent an attempt to encourage a University management style and culture in which recognition of and respect for all members of its community is the paramount value and where a climate of genuine trust, participation in decision making and collaboration is fostered. The assumption then is good and fair ethical practice will naturally evolve and become the norm . . .
>
> (Henry *et al.*, 1992 p32)

Part Two of the EVA Report introduces ways in which an ethics audit may be carried out. Six methods of data collection were used. These included a questionnaire, an open ended interview technique, a values identification grid, case studies through an ethics hotline, analysis of policies and a curriculum analysis (see Appendix 1). The sample of respondents for the research project was selected on a non-experimental basis. The research team made a conscious decision to utilise several methods for collecting data, in order to validate and encourage credibility to the exploratory study. The principles of confidentiality and anonymity were of paramount importance in order to protect those respondents who participated in the project. A total of 603 members of staff participated in the ethics audit out of a total of 1200.

Wilson (1993) states that an audit's methods involve moving from mission statements and codes through to examining the way in which an organisation supports and nurtures its values. It may be relevant, therefore, to give a brief summary of the organisation's policy analysis. It seemed impossible to complete a policy analysis of all the organisational policy documents because of the time restriction in carrying out the audit, therefore selective policies were chosen that seemed highly relevant and important for the nurturing of the organisation's values. It was stated at the outset that staff ought to familiarise themselves with the organisational policies and that a process of continual review ought to occur in order to monitor changes. The organisation did have a specific policy on ethics and an ethics committee. It was advised that the ethics policy be revised to include a more active role of the ethics committee, addressing issues of both professional behaviour and research practice. The findings from both the interview and case study data indicated that an organisational code of professional practice ought to be constructed which would support both research and management practice. One respondent clearly stated: 'I think it is paramount that we research and we research properly but we must research ethically' (Henry *et al.*, 1992 p29).

The organisation obviously had a policy of equal opportunities and it involved removing unfair discriminatory practices. Whilst the organisation, to its credit, had developed a good framework for recognising the importance of equal opportunities and the policy analysis supported the idea of continuous review, the equal opportunities committee should be more active with specific roles identified. It was necessary to further develop a coherent framework in which to operationalise policy. The findings from the data reflected a need to improve the 'psychological feel' or climate of the organisation to ensure fair and just treatment. Most case study data related to individuals' dissatisfaction with their treatment.

Other policies which had been chosen for analysis were the organisation's policies of openness, research, sexual harassment and training and development, all of which needed continuous review and modification. Other policies such as disability and special needs were equally as important, and if time had permitted, would have been part of the 'in-house' ethics audit.

Part Three focuses upon major principles that are essential to applied ethical theory. The principles of autonomy, non-maleficence, beneficence and justice are debated and shown to be closely related to the principle of respect for persons. There is a discussion on defining ethics and values. This validates the process as a values audit firmly locked into an applied ethical system for practice. Part Three attempts to formulate the theoretical framework that underpins the audit.

> Values encompass not only morality but political, social, economic and aesthetic aspects of life.
>
> (Henry *et al.*, 1992 p109)

Values are central to a society's culture, attitudes and behaviour and involve individual personalities as well as groups. Whilst values embrace a diversity in commonsense everyday language, the words values and morals are used to mean the same. The EVA takes the position that moral values refer to modes of behaviour and held or shared values. Valuing in contrast actually captures the idea of both knowing and doing. The EVA was, and is, concerned with how we think about and act towards others and how features of the environment, including other people's behaviour influence individual, professional and organisational thought and behaviour. It is hopefully self-evident that moral values, or the process of valuing concern, thought and action and the notion of self-reflection provide the impetus for ethical analysis and debate. Ethics by definition assesses the ways in which we behave and both valuing and those values that we hold. The EVA Project also identified what may be called instrumental values such as 'self-affirmation' and 'competence'. These values may not be directly seen as moral values but nevertheless are still within an ethical framework, in that if they are influenced by poor communication or bad management strategies, levels of 'competence' and aspects of self-affirmation will be affected. Exploring the community, individual and group values gives not only a picture of an organisation's culture but also a profile of what the potential development for that organisation might be.

An organisation is the sum total of the values and beliefs of the individuals who work within it endowing a hollow structure with life and meaning. In many ways because of the individuality and diversity of the people working within the organisation, it is also a community reflection of society. Raising levels of ethical awareness and what constitutes good practice is essential for both the professional and the organisation. Charters, mission statements and codes will not solve moral dilemmas but one of their functions involves raising levels of ethical awareness and hopefully encouraging ethical practice. Beyerstein (1993) remarks that codes serve important functions and that moral dilemmas can often be resolved by recourse to moral theory.

Whilst an EVA is, at least in part, the beginning of a process that can be applied to professionals and their organisations in order to access practices, it is also driven by an ethical approach underpinned by professional ethics.

> We'll raise it there's no other choice
> We'll raise it and from foundation to roof
> We'll build a new and decent house
> In which we shall live like human beings
> (Talat Sait Halman in Henry et al., 1992, p38)

References

Apps, J. (1993) Nursing education and practice. *Journal of Advances in Health Care*, **2(3)**, 47–50.

Bellah, A. (1985) *Habits of the Heart. Individualism and Commitment to American Life*. Berkeley University Press, Berkeley, USA.

Beyerstein, D. (1993) The functions and limitations of professional codes of ethics. In *Applied Ethics; A Reader*, E.R. Winkler, J.R. Coombes (eds), pp.416–25. Blackwell Scientific Publications, Oxford.

Department of Health (1991) *The Patient's Charter*. HMSO, London.

Henry, C., Drew, J., Anwar, N., Campbell, G., and Benoit-Asselman, D. (1992) *The EVA Project: The Ethics and Values Audit*. University of Central Lancashire, Preston.

Heywood Jones, I. (1990) *The Nurse's Code*. Macmillan, London.

Wilcox, J.R. & Ebbs, S.L. (1992) *The Leadership Compass. Values and Ethics in Higher Education*. George Washington University, Washington DC.

Wilson, A. (1993) Translating corporate values into business behaviour. *Business Ethics European Review* **2**, 103–5.

Editor's note to Chapter 5

The scene has been set: professional ethics has been defined, what is meant by organisational change has been clarified. Chapter 4 has introduced the EVA as a means whereby these two concepts can have a working relationship. Now in Chapter 5 we see the first portrait painted of how the EVA can work in practice.

No values audit will be commissioned in an organisation without managerial support and authority. Here we see the EVA as a managerial instrument of change. It is offered as an ethical structure underpinned by the theory portrayed particularly in Chapters 1 and 4 by which management can effect change.

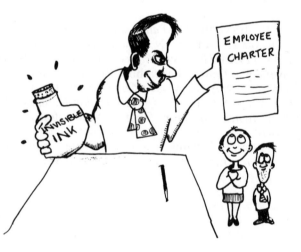

5 The ethics of an organisation

Glenys Pashley

Higher education (HE), like other sectors of the public services such as health care, is undergoing change brought about through legislative, political, economic and social pressures. This demand for change is seen to be necessary for HE and health institutions in order to become, for example, more accountable, to provide value for money and evidence of improved quality. This element of externally driven change can be contrasted with a source of change which is internally generated. Internal change may arise because of a perceived need for restructuring an organisation. Internal change could also be instigated due to the numerous and diverse moral issues currently coming to the fore in relation to an institution's activities, for example, the issue of whistle blowing, discriminatory practices and dishonesty. It could be argued there is a connection between externally and internally driven change, in the sense that an improvement in the ethical behaviour of a workforce within an organisation can work to enhance effectiveness, accountability and quality. Acknowledgement of this connection may well serve to emphasise that 'higher' levels of codes of ethics or ethical behaviour adopted by an organisation can be in the self-interest of that organisation. It is argued here that an emphasis upon ethical behaviour within a strong corporate culture can be strategic for organisational survival and success.

An important and dominant concept in current thinking is the idea of a corporate culture. The virtue of this concept lies in its social emphasis and rejection of 'atomistic individualism'. It acknowledges people as fundamental to the organisation, openly embraces the idea of ethics and recognises that shared values hold a culture together. The ethical dimension is increasingly seen as an integral aspect of organisational culture. A strong organisational culture has the potential to provide structure, standards and a values system in which individuals can operate.

It could be argued that ethics often comes down to personal decisions and that those decisions ultimately affect the corporate image of the organisation (and the culture). Epstein (1987) proposes that business ethics is essentially concerned with the value-based individual and organisational reflection and choice regarding the moral significance of personal and corporate actions. However, Stone (1975) argues that when individuals are placed in an organisational structure some of the ordinary internalised constraints (or anti-social behaviour) seem to loose their hold. He concludes by suggesting that organisational life is construed by participants as 'play' rather than as having anything of morality. According to Raiborn and Payne (1990), the corporate culture of an organisation impacts significantly on the behaviour of the employees. Several research studies reviewed by Frederick (1988) found that individuals, particularly at executive and middle manager levels, felt that there was pressure to conform to organisational standards and often found that they had to compromise personal principles. Frederick concluded that the real problem of unethical behaviour rests not with individual employees but with the organisation's culture and climate and found that even the most upright people are apt to become dishonest and unmindful in their civic responsibilities when placed in a typical corporate environment. According to Kelly (1988), the term 'destructive achievers' has been coined to refer to those managers who sacrifice ethics, organisational effectiveness and benefits to the group in favour of efficiency, short-term results and personal power and success. Such destructive achievers are held to threaten any commitment to social values and ethics and to those managers who do in fact attempt to nurture and encourage a culture of practical ethics.

The moral issues currently deriving from organisational activity seem to suggest that change is indeed needed. An important point to raise is whether change in the individual will lead to change in the organisation or vice versa. Shaw and Barry (1992) discuss the problems surrounding two of the roles that a significant number of people must reconcile. First is the role of the private individual; generally a decent responsible person needing moral principles. Second is the role of the individual as a member of an organisation; generally a person who rarely exhibits or is expected to exhibit any of the moral sensitivity usually attributed to the private individual. This distinction of roles implies that an individual is unlikely to experience shared moral ground between personal and organisational values and that more often than not, conflict will be the result. Organisational values tend to dominate, hence the private individual is usually expected to repress personal values. It may well be the case that private individuals prefer to be morally responsible, as opposed to conscienceless team players. However, organisations tend to require that employees adhere to organisational norms and encourage commitment and conformity to these. In other words, the role of the individual as a member of an organisation will come to define the individual, rather than the private individual defining the organisational role. This is best illustrated when consideration is given to the whistle blower – an individual who steps out of the organisational role. This person generally faces difficulties, including that of isolation.

It is acknowledged that in organisational practice there are few circumstances in which a solitary solution provides for the best action. Nevertheless, Ruggiero (1973) isolated three aspects common to all ethical systems: obligations, ideals and effects. In an organisational context a useful approach to moral questions will involve:

1. the obligation that derives from organisational relationships;
2. the ideals involved;
3. the effects or consequences of alternative actions.

According to Ruggiero, an action that honours obligations, advances ideals and benefits people can be presumed to be moral. An action which does not meet any one of these criteria can be considered as morally suspect.

An important question at this point is, what kind of action can be considered as morally suspect within an HE institution or in a health care organisation? To approximate towards any kind of answer to this question an ethics and values audit would be the first step; that is, an understanding of the culture within an organisation that impacts upon the behaviour of individuals. As Wilcox and Ebbs (1992a) suggest, a values audit is one way of assessing the discrepancy between explicit and implicit values. A values audit should not be seen as an end in itself but as a 'catalyst' for further ethical analysis. A values audit can serve to:

- test the culture for its readiness to change;
- enhance greater self-consciousness about the culture of an organisation;
- reveal the dominant values and those of various subcultures.

They go on to identify a values audit as a critical investigation of the ethics of the ethos within an institution (Wilcox and Ebbs 1992b). Similarly, Smith (1984), cited by Wilcox et al, claims that a values audit can foster a sense of community because it highlights the shared culture or systems of values as well as conflicts in values.

When an organisational culture is strong people know what is expected of them and they understand how to act and decide in particular circumstances (Thompson, 1990). According to Fisher, Tack and Wheeler (1988), cited by Wilcox and Ebbs (1992b), shared values (derived from the mission statement) can be argued to foster strong feelings of personal effectiveness, promote high levels of loyalty to the institution, facilitate consensus about organisational goals, encourage ethical behaviour and promote strong norms about working hard and caring.

The Ethics and Values Audit was carried out by the University of Central Lancashire over a six month period from March to September 1992. It was the first in-house, research based audit to be carried out in the UK. The question central to the EVA Project was, 'Do we practise what we preach?'. Wilson (1993) is correct in his claim; the EVA Project examines both the values underpinning the organisation's mission statement and the values and beliefs of individuals within the University. It attempts to show to what extent these two sets of values match or are shared and makes a number of recommendations aimed at achieving a greater synthesis between what is preached and what is practised. It is worth emphasising at this point that the initial process of an ethics and values audit can be applied to any 'people organisations', for example health care trusts.

The lack of a sense of shared values that give direction and purpose is a major problem facing higher education institutions and health care organisations. A seemingly popular solution by many organisations to the perceived absence of value consensus is the introduction or imposition of an ethics policy or code of ethics. From the literature available, certainly within the UK, the formulation of ethics policies or codes of ethical behaviour appear to have been compiled without the necessary kind of analysis to discover why value consensus is absent or value conflict is evident. The EVA Project addressed this issue and went some way in trying to understand the value basis of the organisation prior to any consideration of an ethics policy. In effect, the Project provided the groundwork for further analysis and development with the ultimate aim of enhancing the University's image as a practising ethical institution.

'The process of identifying and exploring values involves research, analysis and debate . . .' (Henry *et al.*, 1992, p2). The audit carried out by the research team was grounded in 'methodological pluralism', the combination of several research techniques. The use of multiple methods allows the investigation insights from more than one perspective and maps out or explains more fully the richness and complexity of issues under consideration. The use of different methods should:

- help to avoid bias because there is no exclusive reliance upon one research method;
- provide information such that each method substantiates the findings of the other methods, thereby increasing the element of validity and the confidence of the research team.

The research techniques discussed below were used as the basis for an introspective enquiry into the values underpinning organisational and individual experiences within the University.

Questionnaire

The values underlying the University's mission statement were identified and categorised as relating to: culture, management, knowledge, autonomy, self-affirmation, images of other people and values. These seven categories informed the construction of the questionnaire. The questionnaire consisted of 62 statements which respondents had to agree or disagree with, according to a sliding scale of six points. The questions were divided into five areas focusing upon: working practices, working relationships, learning and personal development, course delivery and income generating activities. The questionnaire was distributed to 1200 members of both academic and non-academic staff within the University; a 35% response rate was achieved.

Values identification grid

The purpose of the values grid was to examine how individuals perceived others in different role relationships with the University. Individuals were asked to give a positive or negative score to the self and 17 other roles, for example, line manager, students, lecturing staff, University visitors, in relation to 12 positive/negative value constructs such as: open/closed, collaborative/non-collaborative, trustworthy/ untrustworthy, respect/disrepect, autonomous/controlled, valued/not valued, moral/immoral. A slightly modified version of the values grid was given to a small sample of students.

Case studies

The audit was also informed by a significant number of case studies. Individuals wishing to make known their values or experiences within the University to the research team made use of an 'ethics hotline'. Individual anonymity and confidentiality were upheld by the team who operated the hotline, but the information given was analysed and interpreted in much the same way as the interview material.

Interviews

Semistructured interviews were carried out with members representing the diverse groups of University staff. The material derived from these interviews was analysed, resulting in the development of several categories. The interview technique yielded a wealth of information that enabled the research team to pursue further an introspective investigation of individual and organisational values.

In support of these four main research techniques the team carried out an analysis of University policies and an analysis of the curriculum.

The information gleaned by using methodological pluralism resulted in an interesting and insightful discussion of practices and values within the University. The discussion identified positive and 'good' practices and values and negative and 'poor' practices and values. As a proactive, creative and functional response to the identification of negative and poor practices and values within the University, the research team proposed a number of recommendations for all University staff to discuss and debate.

Recommendations of the EVA Report

It was suggested that leadership within the University involve a more personal and visible approach and that this would go some way towards staff feeling more valued and promoting a shared understanding of the different pressures under which both management and staff have to work.

A recommendation was made that management adopt and commit themselves to the very positive 'charter for management' which was developed earlier by a University working party. The charter for management embodies and promotes such values as: respect, openness, honesty, trust and collaboration.

The development of a caring and collaborative culture was thought to be necessary and that this ought to be fostered through more effective leadership.

The University's mission statement ought to be more precise and so focused that it can easily be internalised by all staff.

It was suggested that a more practical use be made of the mission statement, policy statements and the charter for management by developing a code of professional conduct.

A person-centred approach to management was emphasised through the recommendation that a director responsible for human resources and internal communications be appointed. The individual would be advised to review:

- organisational communication;
- staff experience, expertise and interests;
- career and promotion strategies;
- professional and personal staff training and development;
- policy statements seeking to enhance values and ethics.

A staff handbook was recommended to include the mission statement, code of professional conduct, charter for management, copies of all policy statements and advice about what constitutes good and bad practice.

As a physical endorsement of the principle of effective communication it was recommended that continued improvements be made to the working environment.

The promotion of a 'learning community' was recommended, i.e. an emphasis upon teaching, broader forms of inquiry and democratic relationships rather than intellectual specialisation and hierarchy.

Two final recommendations focus on the carrying out of an ethics and values audit involving students and an audit of values in the curriculum.

Underpinning the development of these recommendations was the identification of several problems which need to be addressed by the University. These problems are encapsulated within three broad headings: 'depressed motivation and morale'; 'delayed decision making and poor quality decision making'; and 'conflict and lack of co-ordination'.

Depressed motivation and morale was seen to result from: inconsistent and arbitrary decisions being made; a lack of delegation in decision making processes; a perception by staff that they have little responsibility and opportunity; unclear priorities in times of competing pressures and an inadequate level of support when faced with work overload.

Delayed decision making and poor quality decision making was held to be the result of: hierarchy which does not facilitate information reaching people when they need it; poor co-ordination of information leading to fragmented decision making; insufficient delegation resulting in only a few individuals making the decisions; and a practice of poor evaluation of previous decisions taken.

Conflict and lack of co-ordination was evidenced by individuals believing they were acting at cross-purposes and with apparently conflicting objectives, and by a perceived shortfall in effectiveness because those individuals who plan do not consult with those who are expected to implement the plans.

Returning to the question which the EVA Project set out to address, 'Do we practise what we preach?', the audit generally concluded, despite its positive remarks about the University, that '. . . at an organisational level there is evidence of insufficient communication networks and information flow, non-participation in the decision making process, dissatisfaction with the provision of a number of resources, potentially disruptive working environment politics and inappropriate styles of management and organisational practises' (p18). Further, it was found that power and role were abused by some individuals operating in a closed culture. This finding contrasts with individual perspectives laying a claim to value openness, collaboration, integrity, responsibility, respect, honesty and trust. This brings us full circle to the earlier suggestion that individuals working within an organisation tend to lose sight of, or are compelled to compromise, their personal principles (Stone, 1975; Frederick, 1988). In other words, the corporate environment within the University leads to a dominance of the individual as a member of the University over and above the role of the private individual as a decent and moral person (Shaw and Barry, 1992). The question arises, are there too many 'destructive achievers' within the University to allow change towards a more caring and ethical culture?

The EVA Project was the University's first step towards transparency, '. . . a testimony to its willingness to face itself and ask hard questions about its values and moral life' (p4). Subsequent moves by the University have been the establishment of a Centre for Professional Ethics. The Centre has a remit for research, teaching, conference and workshops and, hopefully, will take the lead in what should be an ongoing process in the further integration of ethics and values in organisational behaviour. As Wilcox (1992) remarked, it would seem that leadership becomes ethical by serving the common good, by being responsive and caring of constituents and by operating within a framework of shared beliefs concerning standards of acceptable behaviour.

Shaw and Barry (1992) ask what can be done to improve the organisational climate so individual members can reasonably be expected to act ethically. Ethical behaviour requires clearly stated and communicated ethical standards that are equitable and enforced. To institutionalise standards of expected behaviour within an organisation, Snoeyenbos and Jewell (1983) suggest organisations develop a corporate ethical code, operationalise an ethics committee and promote ethics training within staff development programmes, particularly amongst management level personnel. They believe their strategy will enable an organisational culture to foster individual moral action. If the University is to pursue this path then it may well be the case that there develops a synthesis between personal and organisational values such that organisational life is construed by participants as 'moral' rather than as 'play' between conscienceless teamplayers and as an environment in which obligations are honoured, ideals advanced and where all people benefit.

References

Epstein, E. (1987) Ethics in Business. Annual Conference of the European Business Ethics Network.

Frederick, W. (1988) Survey examines corporate ethics policies. *Journal of Accountancy,* **February** 16.

Henry, C., Drew, J., Anwar, N., Campbell, G. and Benoit-Asselman, D. (1992) *The EVA Project: The Ethics and Values Audit*. University of Central Lancashire, Preston.

Kelly, C.M. (1988) *The Destructive Achiever: Power and Ethics in the American Corporation*. Addison-Wesley, New York.

Raiborn, C.A. & Payne, D. (1990) Corporate codes of conduct: a collective conscience and continuum. *Journal of Business Ethics*, **9**, 879–89.

Ruggiero, V.R. (1973) *The Moral Imperative*. Alfred Publishers, New York.

Shaw, W.H. and Barry, V. (1992) *Moral Issues in Business*. Wadsworth, California.

Snoeyenbos, M. and Jewell, D. (1983) Morals, management and codes In *Business Ethics*, Buffalo, New York. M. Snoeyenbos, R. Almeder, J. Humber (eds).

Stone, C.D. (1975) *Where the Law Ends*. Harper & Row, New York.

Thompson, J.L. (1990) *Strategic Management*. Chapman & Hall, London.

Wilcox, J.R. and Ebbs, S.L. (1992a) Promoting an ethical climate on campus: the values audit. *NASPA Journal*, **29(4)**, 253–60.

Wilcox, J.R., Ebbs, S.L. (1992b) *The Leadership Compass: Values and Ethics in Higher Education*. George Washington University, Washington DC.

Wilson, A. (1993) Translating corporate values into business behaviour. *European Review*, **2(2)**, 103–5.

Editor's note to Chapter 6

The arguments of Chapters 4 and 5 are equally applicable to health or to higher educational change using EVA as an example, which was of course carried out in a higher education establishment. The next chapter is firmly rooted in education.

Concentration in this book has so far been on the people who work in organisations either as manager or employee. Here space has been found to mention the customers of education, namely the parents of younger students or students themselves if 'mature'. The earlier concern with codes and charters is continued with regard here to the parent's charter.

The chapter compares the use of values in the EVA with uses in the new theories of education.

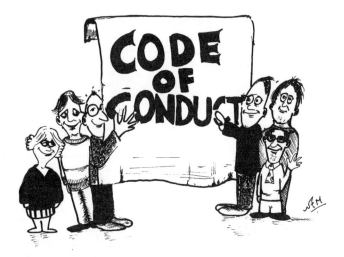

6 Higher education and values

Mairi Levitt

Introduction

In recent years the concern over societal values and the role of the education system in transmitting those values has been directed particularly at schools. Since such concern arises after a perceived breakdown of social order, exemplified by an increase in recorded crime or hooliganism, it is not surprising that higher education has not yet been the focus of attention. Those proceeding to higher education are, *ipso facto*, the academically successful, whereas it is the school drop-out, the truant and the unskilled school leaver who are seen as potential threats to social order. When higher education was for a small elite, both students and lecturers were assumed to share a common set of values derived from a shared social and educational background. The old universities remained largely apart from the changes in access in the 1980s; the 20% increase in full time students was mainly within the polytechnics and colleges, as was the increased proportion of mature students (Macfarlane, 1992). However, the Further and Higher Education Act of 1992 lessened the divisions between higher education sectors, as polytechnics and major colleges gained greater autonomy through the abolition of the CNAA and through having degree-awarding status. The costs of the expansion of higher education fall on both staff and students through the gradual replacement of grants by student loans, the drive for efficiency combined with increased student numbers and new measures of 'quality'.

Openness, diversity and choice

Changes in school education have been justified by evoking the principles of openness, variety and choice. Today schools must publish examination results and truancy figures, provide information booklets and annual reports. Within the state sector provisions for schools to become grant maintained and for all schools to manage their own budgets are two provisions aimed at encouraging variety. Whatever the reality, parents are encouraged to see themselves as consumers with choice over their children's education. The Parent's Charter states 'This is your Charter. It will give new rights to you as an individual parent, and give you personally new responsibilities and choices' (DES, 1991, p1). In the Charter for Higher Education, students, employers and those living and working around universities and colleges are addressed as 'the customers of higher education' by the Education Secretary (DFE, 1993, p1). The themes of openness, diversity and choice have their parallels in higher education with more open access (i.e. to students who gain entry without standard 'A' levels), diversity of courses and greater student choice through modular schemes. The widening of access in itself need not change the nature of higher education courses nor guarantee equal opportunities once students have been admitted (Kearney and Diamond, 1990). However, the development of mission statements, equal opportunities policies and other public statements of common purposes have opened up a discussion of shared values in an area where they had been taken for granted.

The University of Central Lancashire has, in common with other educational organisations, produced an equal opportunities policy which refers to widening access, a fair distribution of resources and the minimisation of discrimination. It has also produced a mission statement which states the University aims to promote individual potential through increased participation, widening access, combating prejudice and eliminating discrimination (Henry *et al.*, 1992, p1). Within educational institutions as diverse as infant schools and universities the principles of 'developing individual potential' and contributing to the local community will be found in policy statements. The purpose of this chapter is to examine the shared values of one university, to discuss how far such values are shared across the whole educational system and the problems for those endeavouring 'to practise what they preach'.

Individual perceptions of shared values

Through individual interviews with staff, carried out as part of the EVA Project at the University of Central Lancashire, a cluster of values was identified as significant to individuals (Henry *et al.*, 1992, p9). The values included openness, communication, collaboration, awareness, being valued, respect, integrity, being moral, responsibility, autonomy. These values can be grouped under three headings: openness, moral behaviour and professionalism. Openness, defined as being 'receptive to ideas and adaptable to change', was seen as essential in a complex organisation (Henry *et al.*, 1992, p70). Being open presupposes other values identified by the staff; that is, communication, collaboration with others and at least an attempt at awareness or the ability to understand others' views. The values which refer to moral behaviour were being valued as an individual, respecting others, integrity and 'being moral' which was defined as 'treating others as one would wish to be treated' (Henry *et al.*, 1992, p73). Finally, responsibility and autonomy were linked to professionalism. To have responsibility presupposes the ability to make one's own decisions and act without unnecessary control.

The values which individuals identified as significant supported the values promoted by the University in its public policies. These values, together with the value of being assertive, were included in a values identification grid administered to a sample of staff and students (Henry *et al.*, 1992 p2). Respondents were asked to indicate a positive or negative score for each of the 12 values in relation to 18 roles within the University. These roles were clustered in three groupings: firstly, the individual, comprising the self, spouse/partner and friend within the University; secondly, the workplace, comprising peer group and line manager; and thirdly, the more distant members of the organisation, comprising the deans, rectorate and University board. It was found that the greater the 'distance' from the self the role was, the more negative was the perception of values (from 16 per cent within the individual grouping to 36 per cent in the workplace and 48 per cent in the organisation grouping) (Henry *et al.*, 1992, p58).

At least 96% of the staff sample saw themselves as open, communicative, collaborative, having integrity, being trustworthy, responsible and moral while rating all other people/roles less positively than themselves on these values. The same pattern was found among students who rated teaching staff less positively than themselves. Since the negative constructs such as closed, non-communicative and even immoral were not attractive qualities to admit to, the positive responses for 'self' are not particularly informative. However, responses for other people/roles did show the way others are categorised as 'like us' and 'not like us'. Thus the responses for spouse/partner and friend in the University were closest to those for 'self' and the responses for 'member of the rectorate' were the most different from 'self' (Henry *et al.*, 1992, p60). The tendency to give positive responses for oneself made the few values which received a higher proportion of negative responses of interest. At least 40 per cent of staff did not see themselves as autonomous, assertive or valued but rather as controlled, not assertive and not valued (Henry *et al.*, 1992, p59). From these responses, together with the interviews and case studies, a number of themes could be identified which drew together the views of the staff and will be considered next.

Positive and negative themes

The positive themes gave a picture of staff working within informal, supportive networks and finding mutual respect and trust in intergroup relationships. Negative themes detailed poor communication, lack of autonomy and non-participation in important decision making processes. Staff expressed dissatisfaction with the provision of staff resources for teaching, preparation and research, including a lack of time to spend with students (Henry *et al.*, 1992, p7). There was evidence of depressed motivation and morale among staff at all levels. The image that emerged is of staff who saw themselves as open and moral in their relationships with others but undervalued and controlled by the larger organisation which did not allow them professional autonomy. The following quotations from the EVA Project Report illustrate some of these feelings:

'[The organisation] is very task orientated, it doesn't take account of people.'

'Staff should be provided with adequate facilities and resources in order to carry out their duties.'

'There is no openness to new ideas, you are put down.'

'We don't know what is going on half the time.'

(Henry *et al.*, 1992)

When identifiying values staff tended to focus on their relationships with colleagues and management rather than with students, presumably because control over working conditions and resources does not lie with students. Central to the University's official policies and to students was a concern to widen access and provide equal opportunities but this did not feature strongly in staff's answers.

Most staff were educated in the elite higher education system of the 1960s and 1970s and their comments on conditions for themselves and their students imply a comparision with their own educational socialisation. Two such examples were the comments on the burdens and restrictions of financial hardship on students, which have increased with the decline in the real value of grants, and the feeling that 'the pressures are to get students to pass [by] moving towards multiple choice questions'. In essence what the EVA Report drew out was a disjuncture between staff's own educational socialisation, which included an assumption of extensive professional autonomy, and the reality of higher education dominated by a management structure designed to facilitate maximum choice for students compatible with resource income. Such an environment, in which students are customers bringing fee income and choosing their own routes within a diverse programme of study, probably requires the adjustment and resocialisation of staff. Such staff are likely to have gained single honours degrees, studying in small classes with students from homogeneous backgrounds. A typical teacher for them was a specialised academic committed to the pursuit of his/her own research. Students may have a more instrumental attitude to their studies than expected by staff versed in the values of liberal education. The Students' Union report stated that '. . . the student should get his or her money's worth' (Henry *et al.*, 1992, p120).

Shared values in education

Within the school sector religious education and assemblies are seen by many as having a role in instilling values. The debate on the 1988 Education Reform Act in both Houses of Parliament revealed high expectations of religious education, not only among the traditionalists who saw it as making children 'good', but also among supporters of multicultural religious education who saw it as a vehicle for teaching children tolerance and empathy towards those with cultures different from their own (Hansard, 1988). Although religious education and daily worship had been compulsory in England and Wales since 1944 the Bible-based instruction in Christianity and Christian worship did not stem the decline in church attendance or lead to an obvious improvement in morality. The decrease in recorded church attendance and Christian beliefs since 1944 made it even less likely that all the teachers taking part in Christian worship would share the Christian faith, although they might subscribe to general 'Christian values'. The EVA Report showed the importance of shared values at all levels of an organisation and the importance of individuals perceiving that these values are practised as well as preached. Some schools attempt to be microcosms of values not held in society at large, particularly schools for a religious minority group, but most educational organisations will reflect shared values within the wider society. Rather than aiming to instil particular religious beliefs all modern syllabuses of religious education seek to inculcate more general social values. An example from Cornwall, where few schools will have any children from religious backgrounds other than Christian, shows that empathy and understanding of other cultures and religions are no longer only for children in multicultural areas. The syllabus aims:

> To create in pupils a capacity for tolerance and empathy, to enable them to live with people of different ways of life, without feeling threatened; to remove sources of racial, religious and social conflict.
>
> (Cornwall Education Committee, 1989, p7)

These values are becoming official policy in educational organisations embodied in equal opportunities and mission statements and in action against gender and racial discrimination, some of these policies being backed by the law. In the school curriculum external examination syllabuses require students to argue different points of view and to try to 'put themselves in other people's shoes' to gain a greater understanding of people in the past or from different cultures and religions. In a report on assessing religious education, pupils who were considered 'less than average' were those who did not listen to the opinions of others, were insensitive to others' beliefs and were unable to share or discuss ideas (Copley *et al.*, 1991, p300ff). Tolerance and empathy were expected rather than any particular beliefs or opinions. The HMI report on the secondary curriculum concluded that in a pluralist society the one value essential to social cohesion was that of toleration (Neal, 1982, p4).

Freedom of expression and critical thought have been basic values within higher education and necessary for the traditional methods of teaching through seminars and tutorials. Underlying the value accorded to tolerance and empathy is the belief in the autonomous individual with the right to make his or her own decisions. A recent study based on a Gallup survey provided evidence for the prevalence of individualistic values (Osmond, 1993). Nearly half the higher education student sample 'strongly agreed' that 'the main purpose in life is to fulfil yourself' and another 40 per cent 'tended to agree' (Osmond, 1993, p14). Entry to higher education and success in degree studies depend on individual achievement, in competition with others, and both students and staff may find a conflict between the removal of barriers to entry which allows access to students from a wider range of backgrounds and the maintenance of exisiting patterns of teaching and learning.

The EVA Report showed broad agreement on values together with the feeling that the individual and those closest to him or her upheld these values to a greater extent than other members of the organisation. It is, of course, accepted that few employees will praise those who hold senior positions in their organisation. In higher education, academic and administrative staff who have the greatest direct contact with students will feel that they have to cope with the numbers and resources allocated by those with less direct contact, thereby contributing to feelings of being undervalued and lacking autonomy. Policies encouraging open access and care for students require staff to teach students and provide counselling and support. It could be argued that the divisions between staff are inevitable in a hierarchical organisation providing differential rewards.

The future?

The EVA Report made recommendations which attempted to encourage:

> a management style and culture in which recognition of and respect for all members of its community is the paramount value and where

a climate of genuine trust, participation in decision-making and collaboration is fostered.

(Henry *et al.*, 1992, p32)

Techniques to encourage such trust and collaboration included personal contact between higher management and staff, the suggestion of work 'shadowing', an exploration of decision making processes and development of strategies for participation, a stress on constructive review of 'mistakes', regular reviews and evaluation of performance standards in relation to policy statements and the mission statement, the development of a code of professional practice and a new managerial appointment responsible for human resources and internal communications (Henry *et al.*, 1992, pp.33–34). All these recommendations could make an institution of higher education a more pleasant place to work in by improving relationships between staff at different levels. However, the changes in the nature of higher education in terms of student numbers, resources and public expectations are not affected by 'person-centred' management.

The staff focused their dissatisfaction at management/organisational level but Marjorie Reeves, in her consideration of *The Crisis in Higher Education*, placed the health and success of higher education in the hands of academics and their students (Reeves, 1988). The enterprise has a spiritual basis, 'a faith in the goodness of knowledge and its creative meaning in our personal lives' (Reeves, 1988). For the world-weary academic this view of higher education may seem far removed from the enterprise he or she is involved in, an enterprise divided up into bite sized chunks of one semester courses taken by students with diverse academic experiences and interests. Reeves referred to a 'crisis of spirituality' among higher education teachers. Although the EVA Report showed that staff shared a consensus on values there was a sense that the responsibility for the higher education enterprise and student experience was not their own.

Conflict and change in higher education

There may have been little interest in values in relation to higher education, other than the publicity given to radical students in the 1960s, and there is a widespread condemnation of anything seen as an attempt at indoctrination. However, those involved in education cannot pretend that any education can be value free. The possible conflicts of values need to be confronted; the conflict between open access and traditional academic standards, between staff committed to research within their discipline and the provision of modular degree courses; between obtaining a good research rating and being an effective teacher of large numbers of students. Mission statements and policy documents record the commitment to developing individual potential, removing barriers, providing opportunities, combating prejudice and removing discrimination (Henry *et al.*, 1992, p1). Following these principles the higher education system will be very different from the elite system which formed the pinnacle of a competitive educational system in which the majority 'failed'. In many institutions the teaching staff have coped with large numbers and lower resources per student by teaching larger groups, reducing contact time, providing detailed notes and photocopying texts in an attempt to give students something like the higher education experience of previous cohorts.

Gintis and Bowles (1981, p48) have argued, from a radical perspective, that the taken-for-granted values of a liberal education failed to prepare students for the types of routine jobs they are likely to enter, since higher education is not confined to those who will become the controlling professional and managerial elite. In the United States they saw the response to this discrepancy between education and work as the vocationalization of higher education, with a stress on occupational skills rather than critical thought and a commuter campus to guard against the development of an 'oppositional youth culture' (Gintis and Bowles, 1981, p48). In Britain these trends are also apparent. Critical thought and 'free space for personal expression' do not fit easily into short courses and large groups. Textbook or 'course handbook' based teaching compensates for lack of contact time and the impossibility of providing a wide range of reading materials for all the students on a one semester course.

A structural analysis affirms the view of the staff that they are controlled and unable to affect change. However, a study of ethics presupposes a more person-centred approach which sees people's ethical decision making as making a difference to the lives of others. While it may be tempting to hide behind a determinist view of the higher education enterprise, a more fundamental reappraisal of higher education should focus on the staff/student relationship at its core whilst acknowledging the structural constraints within which the relationship must operate. The work of lecturing staff must be more than a matter of helping students to get through a series of assessment hoops.

References

Copley, T., Priestley, J., Wadman, D. and Coddington, V. (1991) *Forms of Assessment in Religious Education. The Main Report of the FARE Project*. The FARE Project, Exeter.

Cornwall Education Committee (1989) *Syllabus for Religious Education*.

DES (1991) *Parent's Charter*. Department of Education and Science, London.

DFE (1993) *The Charter for Higher Education*. Department for Education, London.

Gintis, H. and Bowles, S. (1981) Contradiction and Reproduction in Educational Theory. Dale, R. *et al.* (eds) *Education and the State. Vol.1.* Open University Press, Milton Keynes.

Hansard (1988) *Parliamentary Debates (Hansard) House of Commons*. No.130, columns 403, 411, 416.

Henry, C., Drew, J., Anwar, N., Campbell, G. and Benoit-Asselman, D. (1992) *EVA Project: The Ethics and Values Audit*. University of Central Lancashire, Preston.

Kearney, A. and Diamond, J. (1990) Access courses: a new orthodoxy? *Journal of Further and Higher Education*, **14(1)**, 128–38.

Macfarlane, B. (1992) The 'Thatcherite' generation and university degree results. *Journal of Further and Higher Education*, **16(22)**, 60–70.

Neal, D. (ed.) (1982) *Spirituality Across the Curriculum*. College of St Mark & St John Foundation, Plymouth.

Osmond, R. (1993) *Changing Perspectives, Christian Culture and Morals in England Today*. Darton, Longman & Todd, London.

Reeves, M. (1988) *The Crisis in Higher Education: Competence, Delight and the Common Good*. Open University Press, Milton Keynes.

Editor's note to Chapter 7

Continuing the section's theme of managing change and still focus-ing on the EVA, the next chapter is based on the role of a character, which is a direct result of the changes which have hitherto been discussed. As the product of change the new educators of health pro-fessionals must both cope with a very different working atmosphere themselves but must prepare their students to work in the changed structures of the health service. The chapter takes up the wider duty of the lecturer towards their students in higher education, introduced in Chapter 6.

Both chapters see the extended role as having some responsibility for the ethical understanding of the student but also for the student's need to function at work with practical as well as theoretical ease. There is need for training in the aspects of the psychological contract referred to earlier. Having its emphasis on professional education, Chapter 7 is mindful that the treatment of principles and values in the EVA are of tremendous importance in the changing professional areas as well. The earlier references to professional ethics find fertile ground for practical application in this chapter.

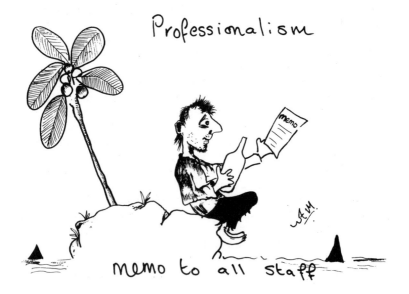

7 Nursing education: the professional educator and EVA

Julie Apps and Margaret Yeomans

Project 2000 in nursing education is, without doubt, the most signifi-cant single factor to affect nursing in 70 years. For those involved, especially with regard to the educational aspects, the amount of change has been of a magnitude barely imaginable (Watts, 1992).

As Henry and Pashley (1990) remarked, Project 2000 is most cer-tainly one of the major policies which will effect change in professional education and subsequently, practice.

In July 1993 a discussion document was published by the Royal College of Nursing, entitled *Working in a Different World*. The report reiterates that over the last few years there has been far reaching and rapid change within the environment in which the professional education of nurses, midwives and health visitors is carried out. Con-temporary approaches to nurse education in the United Kingdom have been powerfully influenced by social and political factors. This is taken a stage further by Proctor and Reed (1993), who refer to the past two decades as being the driving force for change, commenting that this has been gathering pace.

The implementation of Project 2000 and the far-reaching effects this will have both in the clinical and educational field include rationalisation of colleges of nursing, with moves which have already taken effect in some areas towards total integration into higher education institutions. To complicate matters, and add to the pressure of change, these moves have come at a time when higher education itself is undergoing major changes in structure and fund-ing. Within the National Health Service as a whole there has been the introduction of trust status and the shift towards a community focus with the resultant separation of purchasers and providers. These far-reaching changes have had a 'knock-on' effect for nurse education, both in the content of the curriculum and in the response to the differing skills and knowledge base required of the diplomate nurse of the future. A fall in the number of students entering nurse education has ensued, although there has been an increase in the size of student groups, in itself a change for those delivering the curriculum.

The advent of Project 2000 has presented nurses with a stimulating and dynamic challenge (Kendrick and Simpson, 1992). As a result of

Project 2000 has been the increased emphasis on marketing of college potential, to provide not only courses concerned with basic education but tailored packages for the wider health care market. The English Nursing Board (1990) recommended that by 1995 all teachers of nurses will be graduates. This has also become part of the policy of the government Health Department and Nursing Division policy (DOH, 1989). There are pressures on many nurse teachers to obtain relevant higher degrees, accompanied by an increasing requirement to fit into a business plan of the institution in which they are employed, Davis (1989) refers to the collapse of the 'conventional career' with a move towards part-time work and jobshares; it is no longer enough to be a qualified nurse, to have a degree and to want to teach nurses (RCN, 1993).

Suffice it to say that the demands on nurse teachers involved in implementing Project 2000 courses are considerable. Not only is there the pressure to increase their own academic credibility, but also the expectation of enhanced clinical liaison, as required by the ENB: 'such graduates should have wide experience, and advanced level of knowledge, theory and research in a relevant area of practice' (ENB, 1990, para 9.3).

The need to enhance quality in nurse education in response to successive NHS reforms and government initiatives concerning value for money moves into the wider public services, where there has been a concentration upon issues of quality in nurse education in the past few years. There is a much greater focus on financial management and income generation than ever before and there is likely to be increased pressure from the government and the regional health authorities to demonstrate the three Es of 'Economies, Efficiency, Effectiveness'. Nurse education, therefore, must itself be cost effective and efficient as an institution, alongside care providers.

At this point it could be suggested there is a fourth E, that of Ethics, which can easily be lost in striving to achieve the other three. In consideration of the latter, what values do nurse educators wish to pursue in their quest for cost effective education (Balogh and Beattie, 1988, 1991)? Values identification techniques seem highly relevant to the staff development and the organisational activities that are needed to establish agreed mission statements and business plans. Questions that need to be asked include, 'Do we practise what we preach. Are we the caring, collaborative culture, as suggested in our business plans and mission statements?' Educational values involve much more than just delivering knowledge for its own sake, what we do, as well as what we say, should clarify that the way we behave towards each other reflects our own position within recognised values systems which can be culturally/socially specific.

The fact that nurse education has undergone, and is still undergoing, rapid and far-reaching change, is therefore acknowledged. Change is never easy or readily accepted, shaking as it does the very foundations of previous stability. For this reason much energy needs to be expended in managing essential change. Kuhlman and Jones (1991), in their discussion of radical change, state that whatever the conditions, circumstances or reasons for change one cliché remains true: 'All change feels like a cock-up during the process of changing. It is only with the benefits of 20:20 hindsight, supported with intelligent foresight, that managers are able to accurately track their progress (hindsight) over an imperfect map (foresight)' (Kuhlman and Jones, 1991). Although the concept of Project 2000 and its eventual implementation has been around for a few years, for reasons not fully understood most institutions have not enjoyed the luxury of its gradual introduction, but have had the changes thrust upon them with little professional or personal preparation. Fulman (1982) however, suggests the implementation of educational change as an incremental process which should take a minimum of two to three years. Effective implementation can only occur, he argues, under conditions which allow individuals to react to the change, clarify their own meaning, form their own position and interact with other implementers in the process of resocialisation, which is at the heart of change. 'The whole climate of change is disturbing', 'nurse teachers felt left out in the cold and were not listened to', are comments typical of nurse teachers subjected to rapid rather than gradual change (NFER, 1991).

Further comment, that change within any culture brings about uncertainty, to some extent compromise and also the development of competitive elements amongst colleagues, may result. Henry *et al.* (1992) in an attempt to qualify this, with particular reference to higher education suggests that, in fact, a double standard may evolve, with a value-laden caring culture being put forward within the mission statement, whereas the reality is a compromise of values both within the fabric and threads of the organisation.

This compromising of values, with the exclusion of the 'fourth E' and added pressures of political, social and economic influences, must be considered pertinent when evaluating the effect of change on nursing education, its input into the clinical areas and its established links with higher education. One institute of higher education, the University of Central Lancashire, has recognised the relevance of the possible effects of rapid change by commissioning an Ethics and Values Audit. The suggestion that one effect of these added pressures may be a decrease in the stability of the organisational culture, leading to the compromise of values, is therefore worthy of discussion. In a climate of entrepreneurship and a concurrent high educational profile, it is also useful to consider that organisations can enhance their professional standards by presenting a high ethical profile and adhering to the best codes of practice available (Moloney, 1993). Byshee (1990) in her discussion of Project 2000 suggests that the two areas of higher education and nursing education should develop a partnership that offers mutual support and therefore creates a positive force for change.

One consideration in assessing the effects of change on an organisation is the view is put forward by the Ethics and Values Audit (Henry *et al.*, 1992), recently released as a report from the University of Central Lancashire. The report has much to offer nursing as we continue in a time of change and it is for this reason the report will be explored in light of the changes in nursing education.

In an attempt to evaluate the effect of change on the organisational and personal values of those within it, the University of Central Lancashire made the brave and unprecedented move (both within higher education or, indeed, within the National Health Service) of appointing an ethics and values audit team. The University was fortunate in that its academic staff of the time shared a wide range of skills, essential in view of this particularly sensitive area of research.

In considering the development of this unprecedented Ethics and Values Audit (EVA) in March 1993, the University of Central Lancashire appointed the team of six people to examine the question, 'Do we practise what we preach?'. The University, in parallel with most colleges of nursing, has an admirable mission statement. Hospital wards' philosophies could be considered similar in their own statement of ideals. These ward philosophies and college mission statements, though setting out the ideals of defined areas, all too easily result in dichotomies of idealism versus reality. One could indeed question the appropriateness of these stated ideals in the light of resulting personal, educational, managerial and practice conflicts, when these ideals are not achieved. The answer, to some extent, lies within a caring, collaborative culture where the individual is respected, with beneficial consequences for the client whether student or patient. Not only should the mission statement be a reflection of the ward educational establishment's service to its clients, but also an important statement of the workings of the entire organisation.

The Ethics and Values Audit (EVA) Project set out to produce an institutional profile of shared values. This involved an exploration and evaluation of the organisational policy in relation to the University's mission statement, taking into account its underlying values and the links between values and practice. In examining the University's mission statement it set about identifying the values underpinning it; these values linked to the universal principle of respect for persons as put forward by Abelson (1977). The areas the audit team considered were: culture, with the ethical and functional values of communication and openness; management linked to the values of respect, integrity, communication and openness; knowledge, with the associated values of awareness, respect, responsibility and values; autonomy, linked to the values of collaboration and trust; self-affirmation, with the values of moral and integrity; images of other people linked to integrity and respect; and finally values with the associated ethical values of respect, integrity, moral, trust and autonomy (Henry *et al.*, 1992). Similar values may be identified from college of nursing mission statements or indeed ward philosophies, where the predetermined values may be removed from the reality of practice. The audit not only examines the participant's views of the organisation, but also examines what is seen as fundamentally important to the organisational stability, the facilitation of the staff and students' awareness of their moral lives and values, in addition to those within the organisational culture.

Furthermore, the Project involved the assessment of the teaching of ethics and values across the curriculum, important to consider in that Project 2000 guidelines state that the student must learn 'to respect the values and desires of the individual patient or client . . . . The student must learn that care is not always "doing for" and "doing to" and the skills do not lie solely in practical activities . . .' (p47). The development of recommendations that enhance organisational policy was also an important part of the project.

In order to collect the data necessary for the audit, focus of the EVA Project was on the day-to-day concerns of staff and students, whose views were canvassed using a variety of research methods. It is evident from the research that within this University (in common with other institutions), individuals value moral behaviour and awareness, honesty and trust (as will be discussed later). If these values are to be promoted by the organisation, they must therefore be reflected in a caring and collaborative culture. The organisation's human resource is its most valuable possession and if this resource is treated with respect the organisation cannot be anything but successful in producing a workforce prepared to strive for the economic efficiency and desired kudos of the said organisation.

It follows then that the recommendations of the Report are important, for in a climate change of this identified need to care for the available human resources will spread the spirit of caring within an organisation, resulting in enhancement not only of the students' education but, in turn, the students' own delivery of care.

The methodology used by the EVA Report team included semi-structured interviews, a values identification grid (which is a modification of Kelly's 1955 repertory grid), case studies and action research in the form of an ethics hotline and the analysis of policies and curriculum. The use of a 'hotline' was felt to be especially important, as it was likely to identify the feelings at 'grass roots level, whilst preserving confidentiality and anonymity, factors which were imperative at this stage.

One of the stated intents of the report team was 'not just to provide a code of practice, but that as a direct result of the project the staff and students will be more aware of their moral life and values and those of the organisation.' Statements like this enhance the view that within the nursing field the achievement of this ideal could lessen the trauma that can result from change, as identified (Henry *et al.*, 1992).

The conclusions of the EVA Report are controversial and it is suggested, not unique to the institution in which it was carried out. Identified within the report are ten themes which serve to give an overall profile of ethics and values within the University. The first four are positive, in that they refer to informal support networks, peer group integrity and respect for honesty and courtesy. The development of the informal support network was seen as important with the respondents identifying a community spirit where the values of collaboration and communication are important. Within this caring culture mutual respect and trust were identified as being strongly linked to the ideology of teamwork and a strong team spirit.

The staff and students in the EVA Report sample also identified the values of openness, integrity, trustworthiness, respect, autonomy, assertiveness, being valued and moral behaviour as important to both themselves and the University. These values are directly related to the ethical concept of 'respect for persons' (Henry *et al.*, 1992.)

The remaining six themes, however, refer to factors that lead to personal and/or professional conflict. The themes discussed include poor information flow, no participation in the decision making processes, abuse of power, changed working environments and dissatisfaction with resources, charges that could easily be levelled at the organisations involved in Project 2000 implementation and development.

With reference to the culture of the institution the report describes it as a 'closed culture' which operates with a 'fortress mentality', which may emerge as a 'coping' mechanism during periods of change. There is also a section on the abuse of power, with the comment, 'Whilst knowledge is a value in its own right, there is a perception that knowledge is used inappropriately to influence decisions and is withheld on the basis that knowledge is power . . .' Within the institution it is perceived that whilst gamesmanship is an acceptable part of organisational behaviour, respect and value for persons becomes unimportant (Henry *et al.*, 1992). On further reading the Report states, 'There is a widely held perception that the University is a community promoting the values held by the organisation. However there is tension between what that organisation appears to promote and the way in which individuals are treated'.

Arygris (1976) puts forward the view that the organisational climate may affect its ability to focus and develop. With particular relevance to nursing and higher education, it is suggested that a supportive climate enhances learning and development in several ways. In contrast a closed or defensive climate can severely limit the possibilities for organisational development, with undiscussed issues and collaborative enquiry becoming difficult. An integral part of a closed culture is lack of respect for persons, a consequence being the non-sharing of information and lack of collaboration, autonomy and openness.

Another destructive feature of organisational conflict is a loss of sense of proportion. The staff in the audit sample perceived that 'gamesmanship' was an accepted part of organisational behaviour, with little respect for the individual as a person. Strategies adopted by individuals in staking out their perceived territorial rights may lead to unacceptable behaviour and increase the conflict.

This former polytechnic has experienced rapid growth and change and this has led to some uncertainty. One staff member told the enquiry team: 'We have grown so fast that the personalisation of the individual has gone and you have an outer shell and no heart to the place'. Again parallels may be drawn between this and the rapid change which is taking place in nursing education.

There is a need, with a climate of rapid change, to examine not only our own values but also those of the institution in which we work, as portrayed not only by the mission statement/ward philosophy but also within the institutional fabric, if we are to move forward with a caring culture and enhanced client care. As Christine Henry states: 'If competition and empire building become the only values in an institution then we are in real trouble. It is not a threat to be seen to be collaborative' (Henry, 1992).

It should be remembered that an organisation is structurally an entity in itself and that certain values can be imposed upon it in terms of its public image and the explicitly stated goals and objectives. However, the organisation is also a reflection of the beliefs and values of the individuals within it.

Parts of the EVA Report were echoed in the NFER Paper 3 (1991): 'A nurse teacher remarked that the implementation of Project 2000 had been crisis management on a daily basis'. In relation to communication: '. . . its too many different things all going on at the same time . . . juggling balls in the air . . . all new things constantly being thrown at you . . . you think how much more can you take'. Yet another respondent felt '. . . it was laying the track with the train coming'.

It is not implied that higher education is perfect in relation to its organisational policy; however, one institution at least has demonstrated that an examination of an organisational policy and the values it portrays are especially important in times of change, of particular significance for the education of those students on ward placements destined to become the nurses of tomorrow.

References

Abelson, R. (1977) *Persons: A Study in Philosophical Psychology.* Macmillan, London.

Arygris, C. (1976) *Increasing Leadership Effectiveness.* John Wiley & Sons, New York.

Balogh, R. and Beattie, A. (1988) *Performance Indicators in Nursing Education.* ENB, Sheffield.

Balogh, R. and Beattie, A. (1991) Defining quality in training institutions. *Nursing Times,* **87(87)**, 44–7.

Byshee, J. (1990) Strength status and respect. *Nursing, The Journal of Clinical Practice, Education and Management,* **4(1)**, 20–3.

Davis, J. (1989) Who or what are lecturer practitioners? *Senior Nurse,* **9(10)**, 22.

DOH (1989) *A Strategy for Nursing.* HMSO, London.

ENB (1990) *Framework for Continued Professional Education and Training for Nurses.* Project Paper 3, ENB, London.

Fulman, M. (1982) *The Meaning of Educational Change.* Teachers College Press, New York.

Henry, C. (1992) *Guardian* Education Supplement, 24th November, pp.2–3.

Henry, C. and Pashley, G. (1990) Carving out the nursing 90's. *Nursing Times,* **86(3)**, 45–6.

Henry, C., Drew, J., Anwar, N., Campbell, G. and Benoit-Asselman, D. (1992) *EVA Project: The Ethics and Values Audit.* University of Central Lancashire, Preston.

Kelly, G. (1955) *The Psychology of Personal Constructs.* Norton, New York.

Kendrick, K. and Simpson, A. (1992) The nurses' reformation: philosophy and pragmatics of Project 2000. In K. Soothill, C. Henry and K. Kendrick (eds) *Themes and Perspectives in Nursing.* Chapman & Hall, London.

Kuhlman, S. and Jones, N. (1991) Managing radical change, cited by Buckenham, M. (1992) Academic and organisational change, in *Project 2000, The Teachers Speak: Innovation in the Nursing Curriculum.* Slevin, O. and Buckenham, M. (eds). Campion Press, Edinburgh.

Moloney, M. (1993) *Professionalization in Nursing, Current Trends and Issues.* Lippincott, London.

NFER (1991) *NFER Project 2000 Research, Interim Paper 3.* NFER, Slough.

Proctor, S. and Reed, J. (1993) *Nurse Education – A Reflective Approach.* Edward Arnold, London.

Royal College of Nursing (1993) *Teaching in a Different World.* RCN, London.

Watts, G. (1992) Implementing Project 2000: the need for evaluation and review. In O. Slevin and M. Buckenham (eds) *Project 2000.* Campion Press, Edinburgh.

Section Three
General principles
and policy

Editor's note to Section Three

The final section is entitled General principles and policy. More than anything the section takes the theory established in Section One and exemplified in Section Two and extends it for the future. In any volume about professional ethics, whether theoretical or practical, there will always be aspects where the ideal is portrayed and the reality acknowledged to fall short of that ideal. It has been mentioned that even the ethical principles themselves are ideal. The task of policy makers in government or management is to manifest the ethical theory of organisational change in a way that retains the aspiration of the ideal but acknowledges the inevitable reality of imperfection.

The following chapters give examples of what can go wrong if policy fails to be underpinned by sound theoretical principles but also hail the endeavour of the attempt at good practice which policy can inspire.

Chapter 8 talks about the theory and practice of policies of equal opportunities. Initially the discussion is universal and theoretical but then the argument is illustrated by a practical and proven example of a real policy at work. The argument allocates responsibility equally to all

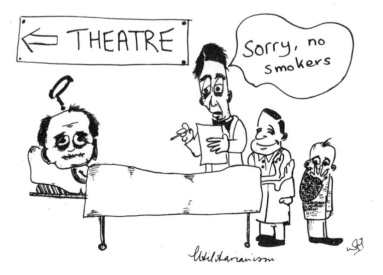

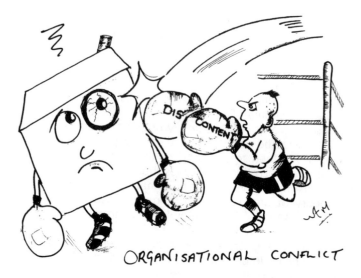

ORGANISATIONAL CONFLICT

participants. Its emphasis on duty and autonomy may be seen as Kantian but yet is practical and the argument has similarities to the synthetic rendering of autonomy, being both Kantian and utilitarian, put forward in Chapter 10 in the context of an ethic of care.

The case studies reported in Chapter 9 illustrate the warnings about policies which may be introduced in an *ad hoc* fashion without proper consultation on cultural values and without regard to holistic theory. The instances are examples of breaches of the psychological contract talked of in earlier chapters. The final case study is the EVA itself which clearly is not an example of what can go wrong in itself but its findings show the presence in the University at that time of, for example, poor communication.

The chapter discusses a practical, organisational, ethical management strategy which, happily, it abbreviates to POEMS.

Chapter 10 takes the health service as a further case study and introduces a theoretical approach incorporating the two major philosophical positions referred to throughout this book and looks at ways whereby they can be merged into an ethic of care.

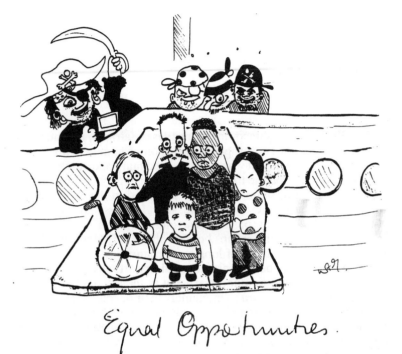

Equal Opportunities.

8 Equal opportunities: the theory and practice

Jane Pritchard

Introduction

In this chapter it is assumed that principles of fairness, autonomy and justice are the right and proper expectation of human beings as persons. It will be shown that when discussing equal opportunity policies, it is necessary to prioritise these principles and it may be the case that a strict application of some of them is sacrificed in the short term for long-term enhancement; for example, strict fairness may not be manifest in policies showing positive discrimination (or, in this country, positive action) to some groups because the principle is subordinated in the short-term in favour of long-term justice.

The best that can be said about equal opportunity policies is that they can be tolerated as a necessary evil in the interim period whilst people address the real problem, namely their deeply entrenched prejudices. Everyone has prejudices, be they about white people, black people, men, women, children, old people, disabled people, people who speak with a southern accent or a northern accent or ostensibly no accent at all. Some prejudices are more subtle; there can be prejudice directed against people educated at public school, state school, single-sexed school or any other sort of school; religious prejudice is rife, not only against different religions but within a single religion, there is very powerful prejudice against different sects. Some people do not trust those with red hair, for example, and for whatever reason allow themselves to be influenced by such notions.

No policy will eradicate these prejudices. The most it could hope to accomplish would be to impress upon people the importance of identifying to themselves what their prejudices are and developing the mental objectivity whereby they are able to set aside prejudice and make a decision based on agreed criteria, free from subjectivity. Agreed criteria of course means something different in every circumstance but, for example, when employing a secretary to work for the managing director of a company the agreed criteria might be that the applicant should be able to speak three languages adequately, have good typing skills, a pleasant manner and so on. The disallowed criteria in terms of equal opportunities would be specifications relating to sex, age, physical attractiveness, race and so on. Likewise assumptions should not be made about the managing director for whom the person will work.

The effective operation of any policy relating to equal opportunities demands that each and every person involved in administering it has a sincere and complete commitment to the principles embodied in the policy. Unless that happens the policy will serve no other purpose than to be a cruel veneer imposed upon a continuing system of prejudice. It is actually more cruel to pretend to have an equal opportunity policy and to go through the motions of adhering to it by, for example, interviewing members of a minority ethnic group, every disabled, old and female applicant and then employing the only white, able-bodied male who applies, justifying the appointment on the spurious ground of 'his more appropriate experience'. It is too often more appropriate to have been, since birth, a white, able-bodied male.

It is cruel to expose people to the hope and expectation that 'this employer might be different'. Likewise it is nothing short of insulting to employ a disabled person because the government says that, for example, 2% of the workforce must be disabled and the company is low on its quota. These are the sorts of results that can be expected if an equal opportunity policy is adopted without the personal commitment of all concerned. Commitment must be coupled with integrity and personal honesty about what 'disallowed criteria' might be lurking either consciously or unconsciously. Unfortunately there are too many people in evidence who, for reasons of their own precarious safety and sanity even, do not permit themselves anything approaching the required degree of personal honesty.

Why then have equal opportunity policies been introduced? Where they have been introduced, what are the principles embodied in them and what means have been used for their design? Are policies written and imposed by management or specified by statute? Is there consultation with those who will be affected by the policy? Does the policy reflect a change in attitude that has already taken place or is the policy itself the instrument of change? What process and content give the policy the best chance of success? An adequate treatment of the topic of equal opportunity requires that all of these questions are looked at.

What are the principles embodied in policies?

The origins of equal opportunity policies lie with the United States Supreme Court's 1954 decision against segregated schools (Boxhill, 1991). This led to the civil rights movement in the USA and from those transatlantic origins Great Britain began to look at its own position. The situation in the USA is different from our own particularly with regard to black people who came as slaves, remained as slaves and for too long have been treated as inferior citizens. The position in this country is not different in principle and in fact, though less readily identifiable initially, has emerged as being almost identical. It is not just a problem for the black population; it clearly extends across all minority ethnic groups. Indeed, some of the arguments used to justify preferential treatment for blacks in the USA, as opposed to others of its minorities, do not work in this country, as really no one minority ethnic group can argue for a different position from another. Historically this country does not support one minority ethnic group over another. Discrimination, of course, also applies to other groups: women, the aged, the disabled and so on. Indeed, discrimination can apply to institutions too; for example, in this country schools are classified as good and bad or at least better or worse. There are categories of universities ranging from Oxford and Cambridge on the one hand to the universities which were the former polytechnics on the other. Just as minorities and women have to try harder to achieve the same as men, these institutions must try harder to obtain, for example, research grant money.

There are two kinds of equal opportunity policies. The first is exemplified by those that seek to afford equality of opportunity to all comers, Boxhill (in Singer, 1991) refers to Justice Harlan speaking of the American position, 'Our country is colour-blind . . .'; by analogy, Boxhill adds that this type of policy should also be sex-blind. Unfortunately such policies, whilst undoubtedly correct in theory and in absolute terms, lack any practical mechanism capable of taking into account the existing imbalance of opportunity. If applied, then the kinds of results referred to in the introductory remarks are inevitable; clearly those with the best qualifications for the job will be, in most cases, the person or one of a group of persons who have been afforded the best opportunity to acquire those qualifications. In both the USA and this country that group is white able-bodied males; it can readily be argued that added to that description should be added 'upper or middle class'. Class is a slightly different problem from race but, as a factor in equality of opportunity, cannot be ignored. Thus in the absence of some 'mechanism' a purist policy of equality will serve only to perpetuate the system in operation before the policy's introduction.

It is easy to describe such policies in operation as 'mere veneer' and to sneer at them; it has been shown quite dispassionately that, as a matter of structure, they are unable to be anything else. In all sincerity and in the furtherance of principles of fairness and equality they should work but because, in reality, there is no comparison of like with like, in this instance it is necessary for the principles of fairness and equality to be subordinated to the principle of justice. In truth any policy will be ideal and will never totally succeed, but benefit can be derived from the endeavour. In this case justice demands the introduction of some strictly unfair mechanism, namely a device to try to redress the existing imbalance: such a device most often takes the form of preferential treatment or positive discrimination.

The two main aspects of the justification of a policy of positive discrimination are what Boxhill calls 'the backward-looking argument' and the 'forward-looking argument'. In the backward-looking argument black people, women and so on should be compensated for the unfair treatment they have received. Thus, notwithstanding the absence of the opportunity to receive a 'good' education and the consequent absence of qualification, these groups should be given the chance to do the 'more desired jobs' and preferred in selection procedures over white able-bodied males who would, without device, have a better chance of obtaining the job, university place or situation. The manifest unfairness to white able-bodied males is regarded as a necessary evil in the attempt to redress the imbalance in society and to change society for the future. In the forward-looking argument introducing positive discrimination, the way is paved for a more equal society in the future. If places at university are awarded to minorities in proportion to their number in the community at large, then it is argued that eventually that proportionate distribution of opportunity will be reflected in a proportionate holding of top jobs.

The theory, of course, is excellent. When the attempt is made to put the theory into practice, immediately there are major problems. One such problem is that there is insufficient unity of control over the distribution of university places to make any single policy reflect the minority distribution in the population. Universities as distinct from polytechnics do not generally have students from a local area. It remains to be seen whether the new universities (the former polytechnics) will adopt a non-regional student base or retain their existing regional bias. It will by now be manifest also that not nothing has yet been mentioned about the personal preference of an individual, as opposed to the group or groups. There are, of course, black disabled women to consider. The policies of whatever kind, introduced for whatever purpose, cannot avoid that slippery slope whereby persons are treated as objects, numbers of this or that sort of minority ethnic group. There is inevitably a fatal flaw of reductionism in equal opportunity policies of this type.

In a discussion of the principles behind equal opportunities it is appropriate to mention autonomy. It must be remembered that any policy will be an attempt at an ideal; there will never be complete equality. It is important also to appreciate that equality does not mean that everyone should be treated identically. If respect for persons is accepted as a worthy aim it is essential that the priorities of each individual are taken seriously. It may not be the answer to insist that as many women as men become engineers; they may not want to. The point is that those women who want to become engineers should be free to do so and will not be treated unequally in their journey along that path. So the interests of individuals should receive equal consideration.

> In particular, the qualifications for a position are the qualities and abilities a person needs in order to perform adequately the functions expected of anyone filling the position, and thereby to enable society to give more equal weight to the like interests of all.
>
> (Boxhill in Singer, 1991, p341)

Autonomy embodies not just free choice but also the responsibility for personal action. A race too can have autonomy. It has at least to be suggested that a policy that specifically prefers the interests of one group over another, far from increasing the autonomy of that group, actually reduces it. It could be argued that, for whatever reason women and minority ethnic groups living outside the place where they are the majority ethnic group must accept responsibility for the position in which they now find themselves. It is one thing for the 'oppressor' to want to make redress or to offer the 'victim' a fairer share but it is quite another for the 'oppressed' to absolve themselves from responsibility. It has been shown that it is fruitless to reduce equality of access policies to so minute a fraction of 'fairness' that persons cease to be individually considered but become numbers. To continue to probe into history for the answer to the question of why this race allowed itself to be oppressed or why women have not done this or that to the same degree as men is vulnerable to the same accusation of uselessness but it is important to bear the question in mind.

Discrimination affects both the institutions and the students who attend those institutions. In the present system in this country 'achievement' is tiered at every level and the ease of passage from one stage to another is, without doubt, riddled with prejudice and discrimination. 'Success' in one tier opens doors to the next set of successes, 'failure' or non-access to any particular tier more or less compels the traveller to take a different road. It must be remembered that what is a 'privilege' to one may be a handicap to another. Policies of all sorts struggle to avoid generalisations about people who, of course, cannot be classified into boxes marked X and Y. It must also be remembered when policies of equal opportunity are designed that their promise or expectation should not exceed the gift of the institution that is itself the subject of discrimination.

That this consideration is necessary raises the question whether or not the rationale behind equal opportunity policies has the right emphasis; rather than give each individual the means whereby they can compete in an unequal system which after all underlines the existing elitism and perpetuates that wrong system of prejudice and wrong values, it could be argued that our effort should be put into changing the way the experience of different individuals with different cultural richness is assessed. Rather than follow some policy of handicapping certain players as though the whole society were a game of golf, would it not be better to stop comparing differences and rating them in terms of the 'norm' experience of the white able-bodied male ('the egg-box norm'). Are we not able to begin to understand the unique phenomenon of each person and accept them the way they are? Rather than put resources into equality of opportunity, perhaps it is more appropriate to put energy into restructuring the society's method of reward. If money continues to be equated with 'achievement' it will never be possible to rescue the individual from the pressure to conform to the egg-box norm. Far better, perhaps, to enable everyone to have a living wage and let personal preference fight it out as to who rules and does not rule in a society which is, hopefully, less hierarchical.

From these arguments what will be abundantly clear is that if an imbalance of equality is identified in a complex historical society it is extremely difficult to put the situation right, even if the inclination to do so is acknowledged. Any policy that is introduced has to be long-term. How such policies are designed and introduced is necessarily problematical. If there is any chance of success at all it will require the patient goodwill and commitment of all concerned. If a policy is overly pedantic or rigid its results will almost certainly be ridiculous. Throughout the long and painful process it must be recognised that it is a policy about people, about persons, and therefore there will be inconsistencies and cases of hardship. With goodwill, however, although total equality will never be achieved, it must be worth the attempt and it must be possible for the process and the results to be perceived as just. Let speculation and theory be put aside and some consideration be given to what is actually happening. The model for this exercise to a large degree will be the University where the EVA Project was carried out.

How are policies introduced and what do they stipulate?

In 1984 the University introduced a policy of equal opportunity. It was introduced by management with no or only minimal consultation with the University (or polytechnic) population. As such it may have more in common with a charter for equal opportunities, being something imposed from above than a code which has the capability of being adopted from grass roots. In essence it goes no further than the legal position set out in various statutes. In practice, whilst progress has been made, and discussion and awareness of issues can in itself be classed as progress, the EVA Report reveals that more work requires to be done. The University has appointed specific officers with responsibility for women's issues, equal opportunities and race relations. The University has recently started holding sessions in 'men's education' where issues are discussed like 'how to cope with male aggression whilst working with women', 'having a female boss'. In addition to its equal opportunity policy the University has other policies, not least of which is its policy on sexual harassment. It has established a multifaith centre. Clearly the University is committed to this area but as has been said, it is a long, hard road.

In research into how many women take science subjects and how many people from minority ethnic backgrounds enter higher education, doubtless the results are used to prove this or that fashionable or unfashionable policy. Whether any difference results from the research or whether the testing has any real merit seems of little concern. Nor is it clear or even likely that these means get anywhere near dealing with discrimination or inequality.

It is not clear whether or not the 'success' of the policies is monitored and if so, how. How this very subjective, person-centric area can be monitored is difficult to determine. It is not suggested that numbers of reported incidents are in anyway meaningful, without regard to an assessment of the individual circumstances of each case. Any static means of measurement of human activity is likely to fail. Human activity cannot be measured like so many tomatoes in a box. Sensible assessment of the success or failure of a policy is therefore a genuine difficulty.

Convincing people to introduce policies is a long way from making them work. It is certain that what happens in the University is likely to be typical of other places where similar policies are in force. A major feature of this type of policy is that once in place it becomes crystallised and absolute. Policies can be used as a weapon just as truth can. Each and every person involved with its implementation must take care that its use does not in itself destroy its intention. No policy which deals with the regulation of areas so subjective as individual behaviour, belief and intention can ever say exactly what the spirit of its creation intended. The policy works best if it sets down general principles based on a sound and sincere philosophical position. Those principles need then to be internalised and used as guidelines to help individuals make moral decisions about particular circumstances. It is when principles are not internalised and the letter of a policy is followed, rather than the spirit, that the danger of abuse of the policy is encountered.

Suggestions have been made as to what more can be done. One is counselling services to look at the effect on the self-image that inequality produces and with it its committal to a lifetime spent conforming to that image. It would seem clear that inequality can become internalised and live on with the individual long after the technical inequality has disappeared. Interestingly, this is borne out by the lifelong 'privilege' of the egg-box norm. To a large degree this feature helps us to understand why equal opportunity legislation is ineffective: it is imposed on people who are already locked into their self-images and continue to behave in accordance with the expectations of those images. This emphasises the long-term nature of any policy and stresses the need for the principles behind the policy to be taken on individually by the people they affect.

Relevant legislation

The legal position in the United States is not the subject of this discussion. It must be stated, however, that it is legal in the USA to have policies of positive discrimination whereas in this country it is not. The significance of that will be apparent in the light of what has been said earlier. From the standpoint that the eventual focus of endeavour with regard to equal opportunities cannot be assumed to be to make everyone conform to the egg-box norm, the absence in this country of such legislation need not be detrimental. Positive action is permitted. This would seem to allow the appointment of specific officers, for example, for women's issues or to look after the special needs of minority ethnic groups, or to give classes in the English language without it being classed as positive discrimination.

The legislation relating to equal opportunities has been well summarised in other places (for example, Chapter 2 of Straw, 1989). The discussion in Arnot (1985) that policies are implemented in parallel with legislation rather than pursuant to it has tremendous immediacy when one looks at what is happening in practice.

> Black people do not want any favours or privileges from education authorities. What they want is to be accorded their statutory rights under the law of the land. If the officers, advisers, inspectors, headteachers and teachers in multiracial areas paid serious attention to their statutory obligations under the education Acts and anti-discrimination laws, there would be no need for separate policies . . . anti-discriminatory Acts already embody the policy on which they can identify their professional duty.
> (Arnot, p11, quoting Gerry Davis, formerly chair of the Caribbean
> Teacher Association)

Thus, what seems to be the case is not that more law is required, and policies, charters, missions and codes can be argued as having a quasilegal function at local level, but that the principles embodied in existing law require to be implemented more effectively.

The position of women is different from black people, of course, as is that of other minorities, but *vis-à-vis* the law they share similar problems whereby existing legislation is not enforced. The position of those discriminated against because of their sexual orientation, however, is quite different. No legislation is in place to protect them; further, the absence of legislation, however ineffective, can be argued to give government endorsement to such discrimination.

Aspects of the EVA Report considered

The central question of the EVA Report is 'Do we practise what we preach?' If we are honest with ourselves, in almost all cases, the answer to that question is 'no'.

> Kant is apparently driven to a dual view of man: we are both phenomenal (natural, causally determined) beings and noumenal (non-natural, self-determining) beings.
>
> (Buckle in Singer, 1993, p180)

Respect for persons is an ethical principle which is an aid to persons in their treatment of others. It falls on the noumenal side and is non-natural. Not instinctive, it requires effort for it to become an operative and certainly dominant factor in our behaviour. If we do not practise what we preach it can be argued that insufficient effort is put in to how the principle of respect for persons is applied. It is assumed in policies of equal opportunity that this principle is acknowledged.

Kant equates the moral pursuit of virtue, which includes the principle of respect for persons, with the rational side of man, the noumenal. Thus this aspect is not natural or instinctive. If it is to be brought to the forefront of man's behaviour it must be worked upon and learnt just like any other non-natural aspect of man's behaviour. If it is true that religious practice has fallen out of fashion in this country, then a sad aspect of this trend is that along with religious practice has gone the practice of contemplation. Meditation and/or prayer or contemplation are useful means whereby an individual considers the theory behind behaviour. It is a sad fact that non-natural behaviour, including the respectful treatment of others, would seem to be readily forgettable even if the theory, when considered, is sincerely accepted. Personal contemplation of one's own belief system and the consistency, or more likely inconsistency, with which it is put into practice is a sadly neglected part of everyday life. It is very easy to think that because theoretical 'right thinking' beliefs are in place, behaviour in keeping with those beliefs happens automatically. It does not. If policies of this type are ever to be successful it is essential for each and every one of us to put real effort into its operation. Natural inclination, and it is hopelessly unrealistic not to acknowledge that everybody has some prejudice that feeds one's instinctive behaviour to be unkind to others or worse, is to ignore them but by whatever means to discriminate against them. Kant maintains that man cannot avoid his inclinations but can choose to ignore them and to do his duty. One such Kantian duty is to act so '*as to treat humanity, whether in your own person or in any other, never solely as an end but always also as a means.*' (Norman, 1983, p102). From this comes the Kantian notion of respect for persons which, of course, reverberates with the maxim '*Do unto others as thou wouldst have done unto thee*'. According to Kant, therefore, we are not naturally rational beings.

The practice revealed in the EVA Report would seem to show that whilst the theory of equal opportunities was officially in place, it was not being implemented on a daily basis by all the members of the community. Elsewhere in this book there will be discussion about how policies are introduced and whether or not they are owned; for the purposes of this chapter it is assumed that if there is a policy its merits are accepted. The emphasis here therefore, is on how it can work. It is argued further that one reason why it does not work is that individuals, and each person is included in that description, are lazy about making it work. Too much power is given to the piece of paper or the law. If it is in place therefore it works is too common an assumption. People also readily assume that it is only other people who are racist, sexist, embarrassed about disability, ageist and so on whereas it is each and every one of us in various different ways.

Summary and closing remarks

When discussing equal opportunities in practice it is very easy for emotions to run high. Let it be said that, whilst passion is an important source of the energy that facilitates change, it also liable to be a factor which alienates the very people, for example, 'those in power', who most need to be persuaded. Those who advocate change and policies free from discrimination, are often themselves the most self-righteous and intolerant. It is important to remember that the egg-box norm had no more choice in the accident of birth than the most oppressed member of our society. If power and privilege are to be redistributed, then those people who have benefited from the existing system must give up power and privilege. It cannot be supported as an effective or ethical method that they should be compelled to give that up; they must be persuaded. As part of the means of that persuasion it is suggested that some understanding of how they feel and their perspective is essential. For example, and this is acknowledged as a dangerous area, a manager in charge of a university situated in an area containing a large number of minority ethnic groups, for purely business reasons cannot sensibly afford to alienate so large a proportion of the 'customer base'. Consequently it is likely that an equal opportunity policy will be attractive to that manager who must instigate it, though for different reasons. Rather than concentrate on whether or not the policy is ineffective because it is not taken seriously by management as an ideal, thereby promoting further disharmony, would it not be better to concentrate on the common interest, namely that both sides want students from minority ethnic groups to come to the university and thereafter to persuade management that it would be even more successful as a management tool if those students were also happy as a result of being treated fairly? After all, word of mouth is the best form of advertising and happy students sell the institution to other people who may become students. By these means, it is argued, cynically or otherwise, that both sides, those in favour of equal opportunity and those opposed to it but willing to utilise it, will be putting their effort into the same struggle rather than fighting each other. There is only one loser in that fight and that is the disadvantaged person over whom the conflict is fought.

References

Arnot, M. (ed.) (1985) *Race and Gender. Equal Opportunities Policies in Education*. Pergamon Press, Oxford.

Boxhill, B.R. (1991) Equality, discrimination and preferential treatment, in, *A Companion to Ethics*, Singer, P. (ed) Blackwell Publishers, Oxford.

Buckle, S. (1991) Natural Law, in, *A Companion to Ethics*, Singer, P. (ed.) Blackwell Publishers, Oxford.

Norman, R. (1983) *The Moral Philosophers*. Oxford University Press, Oxford.

Straw, J. (1989) *Equal Opportunities: The Way Ahead*. Institute of Personnel Management, London.

Editor's note to Chapter 9

Both Chapter 8 and Chapter 9 show the success and failure of policies as they can apply in practice. They exemplify the central theme of the book, namely, theory in practice.

Chapter 8 sets out the theory operating behind equal opportunities, the only place where such policies are discussed. Chapter 9 is able to draw on the earlier theoretical and practical discussion as it is centred in the EVA.

Chapter 9 takes the theme of this section by putting forward a strategy whereby policy can be made to avoid some of the pitfalls of organisational change which the EVA reported.

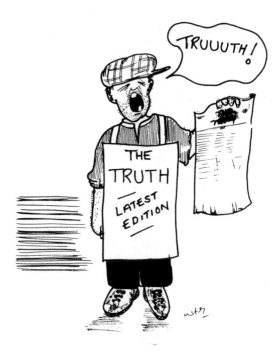

9 Mismatch of policy and practice

Christine Henry

It is often the case that when organisations are subjected to external political and economic pressures that demand change, the internal management of change is often termed as crisis management. According to Bellah *et al.* (1985), there seems to be a plethora of new charters and codes when a culture itself is undergoing change. This development of charters and codes may also occur because there is some evidence for a lack of consensus of values within society generally. This chapter attempts to outline some of the findings from the EVA. Some specific organisational case studies will be discussed and the EVA itself generally will be perceived as a management case study. Finally there is a discussion of an internal management strategy that may improve the management of change within the organisation.

Organisational perspectives

Shared values, shared goals and activities will obviously contribute to the quality of working relationships and the successful outcome for the organisation. Never more so than now must both health and educational organisations seriously attempt to manage the changes effectively in order to improve their service to society. Furthermore, they must develop flexible management strategies and organisational policy that will prepare them for future changes and developments, as we move into a new and changing system of ideas for the year 2000. It is important to go forward taking a more optimistic approach rather than continually 'groaning' about the inevitable change and perhaps to some extent mismanagement. An organisation's most valuable possession is its human resources and if persons as members of the organisation are treated with respect, the organisation cannot be anything but successful.

White (1987) remarks that management theory is developed in order to achieve better running of institutions. Management theory or strategy is not a morally neutral endeavour although some theorists may conceive themselves to be morally neutral characters in that their skills are utilised in order to achieve a successful outcome by efficient means (White, 1987). Implicit within the organisational management of human resources is the crucial acknowledgement that individuals will be motivated and devote energy to the organisation if there is respect and value for the individual by those who manage. There is a psychological contract between employer and employee which is not explicitly known or discussed. This psychological contract is very important for those members of an organisation that may be perceived publicly as a 'caring' organisation, where the purpose is to deliver 'care'. Both health and educational organisations are the most obvious contenders. The psychological contract relates to expectations, attitudes, self-esteem, self-value, loyalty, respect and opportunities, all values that ought to be implicit in the caring organisation's purpose. These values all impinge on an individual's willingness to work and make personal sacrifices for the organisation. If the organisation's attitude does not match the expectations and the commitment to its purpose and if members of the organisation are demoralised in that their role within the organisation is not valued, then psychological energy and willingness to work and their co-operation will be withdrawn. Breaches of the psychological contracts cause intense emotions that are often not articulated and may be directed or diverted towards negotiations with formal contractual agreements. Unrest and dissatisfaction occurs, with the inevitable accusations of abuse of power and poor management. The management strategists and the managers themselves ignore the psychological needs and the contracts at their own peril. The results of not recognising the psychological contract involve a downward spiral of misunderstandings and non-communications, resulting in endless conflicts. Managers who therefore presume that their skills are morally neutral are not realistically aware of the value-laden human resource issues that are crucial to the organisation's success. To be an effective manager requires some understanding and recognition of values. MacIntyre (1981) remarks that 'effectiveness' is not morally neutral. He points out that 'effectiveness' is inseparable from human existence and is a necessary part of persons complying and behaving in a particular way. Scheffler (1985) remarks that managers must not impose their own values on others but must acknowledge human dignity. Scheffler emphasises a central management strategy by the recognition of human dignity as an ideal policy.

The psychological contract, when recognised and upheld, holds values that may be termed in part 'instrumental'. These personal qualities of self-esteem and value are instrumental in that they are valuable in achieving the organisation's goals. However, they are not only valuable to the organisation for that purpose alone. Respect and dignity in an organisational setting are essential for psychological well-being generally. Any organisation undergoing rapid change and development will face difficulties and these may be exacerbated by the ways in which ensuing problems are addressed. What follows are four specific issues that may occur in any caring organisation. These four examples may be perceived as case studies and in the following section ways of resolving these problems will be examined in the discussion of an ethical management strategy for the organisation.

Case study 1

There is a personality conflict between an employee and the line manager. The behaviour of the line manager is inappropriate in that the employee is continually being victimised at meetings and in a work situation in front of both clients and colleagues. There are inappropriate memos being sent back and forth. The employee is showing signs of inappropriate behaviour by attempting to manipulate peer group support and showing signs of stress in carrying out her professional work; neither the line manager nor the employee can be reallocated.

It is clearly a management problem and other colleagues must, in some sense, be affected by the situation. How can the conflict be resolved? In reality often this situation may not be dealt with at all resulting in one person being absent from work and/or eventually leaving .the organisation. Levels of accountability are not often recognised, except that the person who is in a more subservient position may 'lose out' in that the manager is not held responsible for his/her professional behaviour. Dissatisfaction may occur with other colleagues but whilst they may agree that unfair treatment is obvious, they may feel they cannot collectively support their colleague in cases where they too may become a victim.

Case study 2

One particular line manager is constantly not available and delegates all their work to the next in line. Consequently, although the person next in line is perfectly competent, they show signs of stress and overwork in attempting to cope with their own job and the line manager's. It has been observed that often the line manager says he is visiting a particular place in the line of duty but is not where he should be. Furthermore, it is known that he also has a private consultancy, although it cannot be proved that is what he is doing in working hours. Do you blow the whistle? If so, to whom? If not, what can be done to resolve this?

Often in the past when a situation like this has occurred, nothing is done, resulting in a build-up of resentment and, in some cases whistle blowing occurs. The person who has blown the whistle, regardless of the rightness of the action and the situation generally and despite moral justification, may still end up a victim in a system that allows for a situation to get to such a stage. The whistle blower may be always distrusted by colleagues and management may regard the person as a troublemaker. To have a charter for whistle blowing is clearly an element of crisis management. Ideally, where management strategies,

policies and structures are in place, a situation ought /
whistle blowing stage. An appropriate ethical manage
prevent such a situation.

Case study 3

Restructuring has occurred. This gives the head of section an opportunity to reallocate some members of staff to different roles. Time
constraints, levels of work and so on leave little time to consult with
staff. Furthermore, senior management insists that information
regarding restructuring cannot be released by heads of section until
agreement has been reached. Rumours in the informal networks are
rife, ranging from fears of redundancy (even though no redundancy
policy exists) to staff being reallocated to completely different
sections. The ensuing level of uncertainty results in anxiety which
begins to affect work, competency and output. What should the line
manager do?

The difficulty in this situation is that often the informal network of
communication is far superior to the formal channels. Furthermore,
there is the unlikelihood of an appropriate organisational policy to
cover such a situation. Crisis management again emerges, where the
psychological contract is breached and even when the real situation is
disclosed, elements of distrust and claims of abuse of power arise.
Working relationships have been damaged and a perception of 'us and
them' arise.

The EVA as a case study

The first Ethics and Values Audit, whilst carried out in a University,
clearly identified several organisational problems that may be applicable to the health sector. In the foreword of the EVA 'Do we practise
what we preach?' is the opening question. Perhaps every organisation
should ask itself a similar question but even more specifically, publicly
accepted 'caring organisations' in both the health and education
sectors have a responsibility to ask such a question. Management of
change initiated the EVA and although the organisation was viewed as
dynamic and innovative, certain areas were identified that raised issues
for concern. (Henry *et al.*, 1992). However, these issues should not be
seen as negative or critically destructive. The audit itself provided a
rich picture of organisational behaviour, a profile of shared values and
some positive aspects of 'good practice'. Several themes identify areas
where difficulties arose. Nevertheless, this gave opportunity for the
organisation to develop a plan of action that has formed the framework
on which to build an ethical management system that may be useful for
other organisations (see Appendix 2). Some areas of concern were as
follows:

There was some evidence of depressed motivation and low morale, insufficient delegation and poor decision making, with little evidence of autonomy and recognition or value for individuals.

2. The quality of decision making seemed poor in some areas. There was evidence of an overextended hierarchy with poor communication, and inadequate decisions and delegation. Furthermore, there was little evaluation of past decisions made.

3. Individuals appeared to act at cross-purposes and, therefore, lack of co-ordination was evident. There was little evidence of consultation and, therefore, a breakdown in planning and implementation.

4. One major concern was poor communication and an unsatisfactory flow of information. This is a problem within all organisations. Research indicates that large organisations can become fragmented and members of the organisation may no longer see or identify the relationship between what they are doing and the purpose of the organisation itself (Argyris, 1976). Alienation may be increased through poor communication and collaboration. Some management theorists point out that persons seek maturity in their work through a degree of autonomy and independence. If given the opportunity staff may integrate their own goals with those of the organisation (Henry *et al.*, 1992).

5. There was obvious dissatisfaction with the provision and fair distribution of resources.

6. There was evidence of inappropriate styles of management and management practices. There was evidence that undesirable 'quick fix' management styles may become the norm. Furthermore, there was some evidence of abuse of power in relation to both status, position and levels of knowledge.

The organisation had already initiated an ethics committee, equal opportunities, sexual harassment policy, a policy of openness and a charter for management. However, it was perceived by some that there was inconsistency in the policy application, which led to the idea that the organisation's public image was not supported by a commitment to policies. This did not encourage organisational integrity. The conclusion can perhaps be summed up by a quote by a member of the organisation:

we have grown up so fast that . . . the personalism of the individual has gone and so you have got an outer shell and no heart to the place.

(Henry *et al.*, 1992, p20)

Practical organisational ethical management strategy (POEMS)

According to Wilson (1993) one method of monitoring and evaluating ethical behaviour is through an ethics audit.

The objectives of the EVA involved producing a profile of shared values, clearly supporting them by ethical principles, examining organisational policy, recommending ways to enhance policies and practices and finally understanding ethical issues and ways to resolve problems. An ethics audit is a process perceived as an evaluation tool and the outcomes help to formulate a plan or blueprint for a management strategy. The first step in any organisation is to look at how things are. One major important action may involve developing new policies or modifying existing policies.

A policy statement on ethics is implemented through mission statements, charters, codes and an active ethics committee. However, the mission statement, charter and code must be clearly grounded in a credible conceptual framework for them to be meaningful. In other words, general moral principles should underpin policy and be understood by those who help construct the policy, mission, charter or code. Whilst a mission statement relates specifically to an organisation and is a statement of intent and purpose a charter may relate to policy and may be applied across organisations as well as within; both will have identified standards and values. Whilst a code provides guidance for conduct and has principles that state agreed standards of practice, it will reflect ethical principles agreed through consensus and finally inform others what to expect, although it does not solve moral dilemmas. However, as Wilson correctly points out, unless there is a model for action that is ongoing organisations must not stop the process with only the production of a code of ethics. A further step may be in the creation of an active ethics committee, the functions of which involve monitoring research proposals, helping and facilitating the development of a code of organisational ethics in order to safeguard clients and staff and creating in-house ethics training workshops. The membership of the ethics committee should not be dominated by one professional group and the ethics committee's terms of reference ought to link with the major policy statements, mission and charter.

Wilson (1993b) mentions that a model for action involves an ethics audit, development of a code, an ethics committee and education and training within the organisation. The outcome of the first ethics audit (EVA) runs parallel with Wilson's model and in addition mentions the necessity for a credible conceptual framework underpinning practice. The following diagram is an example of a practical organisational ethics management strategy (abbreviated to POEMS). This model is a result of the EVA and the action taken in addressing some of the ethical issues and concerns.

POEMS An ethical management system

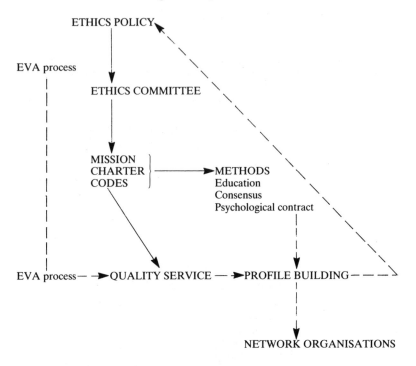

References

Argyris, C. (1976) *Increasing Leadership Effectiveness*. John Wiley & Sons, New York.

Bellah, R.N., Madsen, R., Sullivan, W.M., Swidler, A. and Tipton, S.M. (1988) *Habits of the Heart: Individualism and Commitment in American Life*. Harper & Row, New York.

Henry, C., Drew, J., Anwar, N., Campbell, G., and Benoit-Asselman, D. (1992) *EVA Project: The Ethics and Values Audit*. University of Central Lancashire, Preston.

MacIntyre, A. (1981) *After Virtue*. Duckworth, London.

Scheffler, I. (1985) *Of Human Potential: An essay in the Philosophy of Education*. Routledge and Kegan Paul, London.

White, P. (1987) *Self-respect, Self-esteem and the Management of Educational Institutions: A Question of Values in Educational Management and Administration*, **15**; 85–91.

Wilson, A. (1993) *Getting Ethics on the Business Agenda – The Role of Research*. The British Academy of Management Annual Conference, Milton Keynes.

Editor's note to Chapter 10

Whereas the last chapter was located in its particularity, though not of course in its generality, in higher education, the focus of Chapter 10 is in the health service. This mirrors the alternating emphasis of the whole book between these two examples of organisations in a state of change.

The chapter comes back to the theory heralded in Chapter 1: using health care as an example, the basic ethical principles are put into practice. Combining the approaches of Kantian ethics and utilitarianism towards the principle of autonomy an ethic of care is introduced.

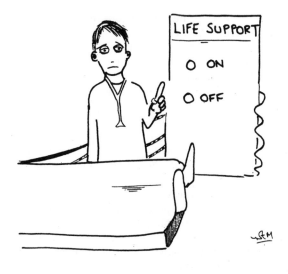

Ethic of Care

10 Organisational ethics: the ethics of care

Christine Henry and Norma Fryer

This chapter discusses issues of ethical theory and the application of moral principles, specifically the principle of autonomy and an 'ethics of care' that involves effectively putting into operation moral principles within the organisational setting.

Applied ethics

The traditional Anglo-American moral philosophy has been viewed as central to both Kantian and utilitarian conceptions and is based upon impartiality, impersonality, justice, formal rationality and universal principles. Williams (1985) remarks that the traditional Anglo-American conception leaves little room for consideration of personal integrity and other broad personal concerns.

According to Fox and De Marco (1986), the challenge of philosophers involves providing theoretical frameworks where practical moral problems may be solved. This challenge occurs from diverse professional organisations as well as in the areas of health care and education. There seems less consensus regarding moral issues and the traditional universal ethical theories may appear inadequate in dealing with modern day practical concerns. Some critics feel that there is a gap between theoretical and applied ethics. According to Fox and DeMarco much of the work in applied ethics takes one particular school of thought and does not deal with the problems of opposing philosophical theory or an existing theory does not give appropriate answers, or in some cases applied ethics is carried out without any reference to theory at all. However, from both a historical and social perspective, philosophers have defended particular ethical theories and argued for underpinning ethical principles that may encourage moral judgement and decision making or act as guidelines for ways in which we behave. One reason that philosophers give in answer to their critics is that if there were no principles for supporting one view as opposed to another, there would be no point in holding a moral opinion in the first place.

However, if we take it that people do make moral judgements and have moral views or opinions (there is an abundance of empirical evidence throughout history to support this), then it seems to be the case that in a social system that obviously has more than one principle, a practical method is needed to resolve possible conflicts.

Fox and DeMarco claim that the changing views of science (science is not value-free) creates not only a new climate of opinion but the idea that if theoretical interpretation of data is important in science then it may benefit ethics as well. Human need, reason and agreement may provide the evidence and give ethics an objective grounding. Hence, perhaps, the need for utilising the social sciences' as interpretative evidence to support applied ethics (Jennings, 1986). According to Jennings both applied and professional ethics are not subdisciplines of philosophy but involve developing ways in which a new kind of interdisciplinary synthesis can occur. Kantian and utilitarian theories and their principles may help to revitalise our understanding of our moral values in a continually changing contemporary world. Furthermore, abstract principles and universal moral rules are embodied in social action and the relationships that we develop in both our personal and public life. According to Midgley (1991), applied ethics and morality relate to the whole of life within both our private and public domains. She remarks that moral rules are central to social and public life and the moral laws of society are of immediate concern.

Principles

Higher education and health care organisations in general may be perceived as 'caring' institutions, simply because of the assumed inherent values within their mission (Henry *et al.*, 1992). A discussion of some moral principles, particularly 'autonomy', may help to clarify the traditional accepted philosophy that underpins professional practice in organisations. In debating a general universal principle a foundation may be built on which to formulate a discussion of an 'ethics of care'.

Ethics as a discipline is part of theoretical enquiry within the philosophical field but it is also part of everyday common sense through our interactions and the way in which we behave towards each other. Whilst principles are necessary for ethical theory they also act as a guide to human conduct.

The use of the term 'person' as a moral term implies that the individual, valued as a person, has rights, is free and responsible and is self-determined and interactive (see Chapter 1). Persons are capable of making choices and through having a capacity for autonomy have an ability for being moral agents. Respect and value involve 'other-regarding' principles and are the focus and guiding principle for 'caring' communities. A caring community may be judged by most as a socially valuable organisation. Respect for persons as a moral principle

relates closely to other accepted moral principles considered important for a caring community.

The principle of autonomy whilst an ideal, relates to having the freedom to choose, being able to carry out plans and policies, making decisions and being held accountable for actions and behaviour. However, in
reality, whilst respect for persons and trusting the capacity to be responsible are essential for autonomy, the individual cannot always act in his or
her self-interest in the real world. Central to this concept of autonomy is
the idea of self-determination and a reliance on individual judgement.
Thus, person autonomy is commonly referred to as a function of 'being
one's own person' (Beauchamp and Childress, 1979). In theory it suggests a person is free from controlling mechanisms and, as Jagger (1983)
points out it is basic to the liberal conceptions of freedom and equality
and will limit the state control. The extent to which an individual is able to
function autonomously is therefore largely dependent on social norms,
values and cultural influences and on any social and political constructs or
measures of coercion taken to control behaviour. In addition, behaviour
may be seen to be controlled when a person's autonomy is diminished
during periods of physical or mental incapacity.

The postwar years in western culture began to see a trend towards
much greater awareness of civil rights which has imposed itself in all areas
of life, not least amongst organisational communities. The emphasis on
rights link closely to the notion of autonomy and encourages more participation in and greater responsibility for decision making processes in
both the professional and management field. It follows that the same
principles of freedom and liberty should apply to any professional group.
A group which is self-regulating and operates through a system of self-
appraisal is in a position to claim an autonomous role because of its recognised independence of action and judgement (Blane, 1986). Groups of
professionals who claim to be autonomous are, however, influenced by
professional requirements that dictate the norms and goals for that profession, a situation that may conflict with or create limitations on personal
autonomy. What appears to cement a professional group lies within the
shared values of its members.

It is clear that the person or group of persons having freedom of
choice (autonomy) must have an attendant right to the choices offered,
a right that may support choosing between competing goods. For that
reason it is important to be reminded that autonomy cannot be applied
universally either as a moral principle or a legal right. Nevertheless
before discussing the usefulness and the difficulties that arise in recognising autonomy as at least a principle to be considered in organisational ethics, it may be useful to briefly address two of the theoretical
approaches to autonomy.

There are numerous authors and texts that examine and provide definitions and explanations of what it means to be an autonomous person.
Two distinctions should be made from the outset. The opportunity to

have choice, freedom and/or a right to be self-determined is itself only an acknowledgement of the potential to be autonomous. Whether one is self-determined because of self-regulatory rules or through societal rules that support human rights and freedom of choice, it cannot be assumed that all individuals have the capacity or ability to exercise autonomy. It follows, therefore, that respect for autonomy provides different ethical parameters from being able to act autonomously in both thought and deed.

Kant suggests that as a rational being a person has the choice of free will and the right to be their own moral agent capable of making independent moral principles that 'can be willed to be universally valid for everyone' (Beauchamp and Childress, 1979). In other words, as an autonomous agent, the individual defines his/her own rules and should not be subjected to the rules and conditions of others. For Kant autonomy is intrinsically valuable, in opposition to the utilitarian view that ascribes value to autonomy only in so far as it is conducive to happiness (Sikora, 1993). Komrad (1983) pursues the view further by identifying how Kant supplements his own definition that we are 'compelled to be autonomous' and that persons have a duty to be autonomous, especially since autonomy is the basis of all other moral behaviour (according to a Kantian view). In the domain of professional practice within organisations Kant's view of autonomy would be exemplified through the notion of his 'categorical imperative' which would 'forbid' even the voluntary and informed renunciation of autonomy (Komrad, 1983, p38).

In contrast to a Kantian perspective, the utilitarian view of John Stuart Mill views the concept of autonomy in relation to action rather than will, arguing that control over individual action is only justified if that action is likely to harm others. The principle of utility allows persons to develop their own potential and ability to judge, maximising in the long term the benefits to society in general. Unlike Kant, Mill would support the view that as an autonomous agent, a person has the freedom to limit the degree of autonomy on the basis that he/she may, by choice, relinquish the responsibility to make a decision in favour of professional opinion. This may apply in both the health care and the educational situation in relation to both clients/patients or students. If such an action has the right consequence of creating a positive outcome, the act would not have been a violation of autonomy. Warnock (1985) suggests that this may lay down the foundation of morality in that an act is right if it benefits the person more than it harms. The same may be said of the principle of beneficence which means to positively help someone whenever necessary. However, whilst the principle of beneficence may be viewed as utilitarian it may conflict with the principle of autonomy (see Chapter 1). Furthermore, beneficence links closely to an 'ethic of care' in that 'other-regarding' issues and the capacity for caring may also suggest interfering in order to positively help.

From a Kantian view it is 'respect for a person's autonomy' that perhaps links closely also with an 'ethic of care'. According to Gillon
(1986) respect for autonomy reflects a Kantian belief in the human
condition acceptable to the utilitarian because it may also maximise
happiness. If the individual is valued as a person and his/her autonomy
is respected and action by others validates the respect for autonomy, it
follows that psychological well-being may be enhanced. This respect
given to the person by virtue of his/her potential autonomy is also
linked closely to an 'ethics of care', therefore perhaps viewed as an
important organisational principle.

Within both the health care and educational field the problems
facing the professionals may well be grounded in conflict between personal and professional moral values, rather than in diversity of opinion
on ethical theories. The professional is governed by the rules and professional or organisational code and an overriding duty of beneficence is
implicit within standards of practice laid down and monitored by a profession. However, there may be times where professional or organisational directives may contravene a personal view held by the
individual (see Appendix 2). It is therefore important to remember
that codes of practice and other professional or organisational directives, whilst serving the function of providing a standard by which professionals should operate, do not provide answers to moral dilemmas.

The power of autonomy is in itself an abstract concept that is clearly
dependent on the context within which individuals are operating.
However, a desire to be self-determined is reliant upon the ability and
desire to make choices, which in turn depends upon having adequate
information to make those choices. It is within the context of ignorance, be that the result of a lack of ability, lack of desire, being misinformed, misled or simply through withholding information, that
members of an organisation may have been unable to maximise their
autonomy. Harris (1991) identifies what he describes as a defect in
information as one of four major influences affecting a person's autonomy. He enhances the view that a person's capacity to choose is
severely undermined when beliefs or values are based upon incorrect
information or a person has been misinformed, kept in ignorance or
told only part of a truth. That is why a poor information/
communication system is a problem for organisations. In addition the
defect may be due to a person's reduced capacity to understand
through a failure to recognise meaning or significance in what he/she
has been told or that the person simply does not wish to know. This
situation seems to be represented within both health care and
educational organisations (see Appendix 2). Other influences
highlighted by Harris include the inability to control desires or actions
where autonomy is compromised through a defect of reasoning where
such a defect is seen as a result of socialisation processes that encourage indoctrination and prejudice, undermining the individual's ability

to make choices. The subservient role of different groups within the organisation may serve as an example. Harris suggests that self-determination improves with time and practice; for some, the capacity for developing autonomy during the formative years is restricted by others who are not willing to recognise how self-determination is nurtured if the individual is allowed to grow from experiences and possibly the mistakes of former years.

In itself the concept of autonomy is an abstract term. It engenders a set of values and respect for those values forms the basis on which an understanding of the principles of that concept may be acquired, acknowledged and supported. Authors recognise respect for autonomy as a fundamental principle employing, as Downie and Calman (1987) suggest, the four moral principles of non-maleficence, beneficence, justice and utility.

Care

Henry's (1986) study on the development of the conception of persons supports a psychological developmental trend that shows we are influenced at a very early age by experience and the education process influencing the sort of philosophical and ethical conceptions we adopt in adulthood. She further remarks that we are influenced by occupational socialisation in the conceptions we formulate which supports the notion that social experience influences our values and beliefs. If this is the case, then obviously the sort of experience we have within the organisation will have some effect on the values and beliefs we have. However, generalisations or predictions cannot be made. Recognising the differences and the similarities in our experiences may help us to understand how we may modify our behaviour in order to follow the universal maxims or principles that guide 'caring' behaviour. One of those major principles is autonomy.

The concept of care as a moral principle may be perceived as a partner or relative (even a junior cousin) of the traditional Kantian principle of respect for persons (Henry, 1992). This does not mean devaluing the moral principle of 'care' by placing it in a subordinate position to the universal principles of respect for persons, autonomy, nonmaleficence, beneficence or justice but shows how, in context rather than in the abstract, the 'care' principle may actually allow abstract universal principles to be put into practice. The danger rests upon interpretation and how the 'ethics of care', if seen as being different rather than related, may encourage a view of it being subordinate. Ethical practice and its underlying theory rests upon similarity and shared principles and values. 'Other-regarding' and caring principles will enhance an organisation's ethical profile and success in the organisational goals. An organisation will operationalise its principles by devising an ethical system of policy and practice promoting the 'welfare' of staff and, by consequence, practising care.

According to McInerney (1992, p152), some philosophers have claimed that the most important issues surrounding morality, rather than general rules applying to everyone, centre on the feelings and concern we have for other people. It may be assumed rightly that ethical practice is equally as important as the underpinning abstract rules and concepts.

A guiding principle and a general maxim is to pursue justice with fairness and to be treated equally. Experiences within the organisational setting may underemphasise care, compassion and the desire not to hurt others. However, generalisation ought not to be made from a particular situation or specific social context, even though it may be that similar situations may be encountered in other organisations where there is a dominant aggressive management culture. The behaviour and attitudes of persons are complex. Attitudes and values are not static and to generalise would be to assume not only that persons may be measured but that they are passive creatures. Furthermore, identifying the differences and similarities in experiences may help us to extend our understanding, rather than offer any sound prediction or generalisation.

The unmeasurable prescriptive generalised principles are more likely to be applicable across cultures. The universal moral principle of respect for persons and autonomy have been conceived as guidelines for how we ought to behave. The traditional western philosophers were persons and shared experiences with other persons in a particular cultural and historical context which obviously influenced ideas and conceptions. However, the present authors believe we make a mistake by enhancing the differences in experiences between individuals within both a cultural and historical framework, rather than identifying the positive shared principles and values between all persons regardless of gender, colour or creed. The ethics of care is an important principle mutually supportive of other principles. It may be seen that, through a philosophy of care, persons as professionals within the organisational framework have the capacity to put into practice those generalised rules or principles that apply to everyone.

If staff and clients are guided by shared values, this will empower and affirm their identity as members of the organisation's community. The values that are shared in both professional and organisational terms must, however, support moral principles. Nevertheless, there may be tension between what the organisation appears to promote with regard to policy and the way in which clients and staff are treated.

References

Beauchamp, T.L. and Childress, J.F. (1979) *Principles of Bio Medical Ethics*. Oxford University Press, Oxford.

Blane, D. (1986) Health professionals. In *Sociology as Applied to Medicine*, D. Patrick and G. Scanbler (eds) Baillière Tindall, London.

Downie, R.S. and Calman, K.C. (1987) *Healthy Respect, Ethics in Health Care*. Faber & Faber, London.

Fox, R.M. and De Marco, J.P. (1986) The challenge of applied ethics. In *New Directions in Ethics*, J.P. De Marco and R.M. Fox (eds), pp.1–18. Routledge and Kegan Paul, New York.

Gillon, R. (1986) *Philosophical Medical Ethics*. John Wiley & Sons, London.

Harris, J. (1991) *The Value of Life*. Routledge, London.

Henry, C. (1986) *Conceptions of the Nature of Persons*. Unpublished PhD thesis, Leeds University.

Henry, C. (1992) Reasonable care: approaches to health care research. *Journal of Advances in Health and Nursing Care*, **1(4)**, 79–91.

Henry, C., Drew, J., Anwar, N., Campbell, G. and Benoit-Asselman, D. (1992) *EVA Project: The Ethics and Values Audit*. University of Central Lancashire, Preston.

Jagger, A.M. (1993) *Feminist Politics and Human Nature*. Rowman & Allenhead (Publishers), Harvester Press, Sussex.

Jennings, B. (1986), Applied ethics and the vocation of social science. In *New Directions in Ethics*, J.P. De Marco and R.M. Fox (eds), pp.190–204. Routledge & Kegan Paul, New York.

Komrad, M.S. (1983) A defense of medical paternalism: maintaining patient autonomy. *Journal of Medical Ethics*, **9**, 38–44.

McInerney, P. (1992) *Introduction to Philosophy*. Harper Perennial, New York.

Midgley, M. (1991) *Wisdom, Information and Wonder*. Routledge, London.

Sikora, R.I. (1993), Rule-utilitarianism and applied ethics. In *Applied Ethics*, E.R. Winkler and J.C. Coombs (eds). Blackwell Scientific Publications, Oxford.

Warnock, M. (1985) *A Question of Life*. Blackwell Scientific Publications, Oxford.

Williams, B. (1985) *Ethics and the Limits of Philosophy*. Harvard University Press, Cambridge, Mass.

Exercise – prioritising

Below is a list of issues and values often identified as important to an organisation's culture. Section A deals with policy and processes, whereas Section B deals with some principles and values. Take the position of a manager or professional and prioritise in order of preference. It may be useful to carry out this exercise within your own work area. It will be enlightening to compare with other colleagues' views and note the similarities and differences.

Indicate which perspective you have chosen: Manager (   ) Professional (   ).

SECTION A – POLICY AND PROCEDURE

A – Equal opportunities policy (including harassment)
B – Research targets – two publications per staff per year
C – Organisational code of professional practice
D – Charter for management
E – Network women issues (resourced)
F – Increasing access to service
G – Charter for clients
H – Separate harassment policy and equal opportunities
I – Active ethics committee
J – Executive management (management in the hands of a few)
K – New in-house training programme for ethics
L – Participative management structure (management shared)
M – Staff counselling/welfare support service
N – Appointment of professor (research)
O – Policy for whistle blowing
P – Research policy of non-animal experimentation
(Total 16)

SECTION B – VALUES

A - Loyalty
B – Trust
C – Respect
D – Honesty
E – Fairness/justice
F – Personal and professional autonomy
G – Beneficence
H – Non-maleficence
I – Accountability
J – Rights
(Total 10)

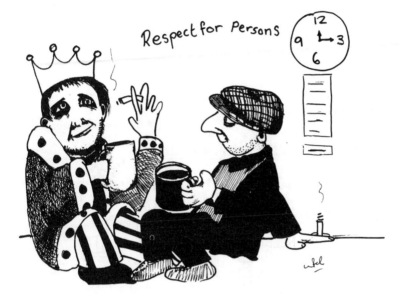

Appendix 1 The research base: the ownership of values

Christine Henry

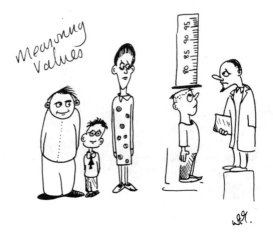

Introduction

This section relates to the problem of how we assess or measure values and some of the methodological issues that may arise. It is perhaps important to ensure that the research approach and methods used to assess or measure values are in every sense appropriate. The research process itself must in the first place be of high quality to ensure ethical practice and act as a guideline for others. However, it is not in any sense easy to measure values. The term 'measure' may have a restrictive meaning and does not easily apply to variables that are in one sense, non-measurable. Therefore, the term 'measure' is used in the widest sense to mean assessing and identifying values. Wilson (1993a) remarks that an ethics audit's methods involve moving from mission statements and codes through to examining the way in which an organisation supports and nurtures its values. Obviously the first step involves identifying the organisation's values then examining policy missions, charters and codes of an organisation. By eventually looking at ways to improve or nurture an organisation's values, methods of evaluation must be creative and perhaps innovative. This cannot be done through managing one or two established research methods and hoping for the best. Before even discussing methods it is perhaps essential to clarify what is meant by values.

Values

Any organisation will have a profile of values and Wilcox and Ebbs (1992) remark that when institutions look towards a form of self-assessment they are required to assess progress through a commonly held benchmark articulated through the mission or value system. However, values, according to Henry *et al.* (1992) are much more subjective than principles and need not necessarily be moral. It is often noted that some organisational values may conflict with personal values. Values generally can have a personal interpretation and may violate or support moral principles. The organisation is also a reflection of the beliefs and values of the individuals within and the two sets of value systems, that is the recognised accepted corporate values and personal values, may not always be the same. An organisation, whilst an entity itself, may have values imposed upon it in terms of its public image, explicitly stated goals and objectives. This is often the case for NHS organisations and the university sector in that the very nature of their purpose is value-laden. According to Bellah *et al.* (1988) values are deeply rooted in the dominant culture and they may shift from one emphasis to another, such as those associated with individualism, self-reliance, independence and competition and those associated with interdependence, responsibility for others, co-operation and community ethos. Either set of values, in the extreme, offer serious risks in that they may subvert the values in the opposite configuration. The dangers are obvious; for example, competition and self-interest becoming the dominant values in an organisational value system.

According to White (1987) the values of self-respect and self-esteem are important. She remarks that policy makers should acknowledge human dignity and find ways in which to give concrete application in institutions. White argues that an authority structure in institutions must enable members to function as moral persons and in this way it will preserve self-respect.

Values are important within both health and educational organisations. According to Wall (1993) the National Health Service in Great Britain was a good example of a service underpinned by a set of values which everyone could share. Furthermore, those people who continue to be concerned in promoting health and education must be still governed by values concerned for the common good. Members of society may feel more reassured if a caring organisation works within an ethical framework. A consensus of values obviously encourages an organisation to achieve its purpose and effectively legitimises the authority of those who make decisions on behalf of others. According to Wall consensus on values has a practical purpose in that it speeds up the decision process. This in itself must be viewed as a useful 'management tool' in times of change. Therefore, it is perhaps essential to find ways of developing an organisation's profile of values as a first step. Assessing and identifying values is part of the process of an ethics audit.

The first ethics and values audit in the UK attempted to explore the ethical dimensions of various values that underpin the mission statement and aimed to identify shared values within a university's community. In addition, the choice of methods allowed for the development of a profile of organisational policies, procedures, structure and culture.

The sample for the audit was selected on a non-experimental basis. The researchers emphasised that the principles of confidentiality and anonymity were of paramount importance to protect those individuals contributing to the study. This must be maintained throughout the ethics audit process.

The questionnaire

The questionnaire was chosen as one method simply because it could be distributed to every member within an organisation. According to Nesbit and Entwistle (1970) the questionnaire is similar to an interview on paper; just as much care is needed in the construction of questions and choice of words. However, the questionnaire is impersonal and there is no face-to-face interaction with the researcher, which allows explanation of the purpose, procedures and possible ambiguities. For those reasons the questionnaire has its limitations, although it should have the same features as a 'good law'; that is, it should be clear and unambiguous.

Questionnaires have to be carefully designed so that respondents do not have any difficulty in understanding the questions and know how to record an answer (Macleod, Clark and Hockey, 1989). The design of the questionnaire can lead to a limitation in the amount of information gathered. The disadvantages are that people often do not return them and there is no opportunity to pursue specific points further.

However, a questionnaire allows for the respondent to record his or her responses from a given set of alternatives, similar to an attitude scale. As a method, it is more reliable because of its anonymity which can encourage a greater honesty from the respondents. Errors are likely to be limited to the sample and the instrument itself and it is therefore possible to get a systematic response from the population in question. It must be borne in mind that the social survey type of questionnaire on its own is not necessarily sufficient as a good assessment of values.

The interview

Interviews restrict the number of respondents who can be incorporated into an audit. Furthermore, the interview, instrument, coding and sample all have the potential for error. The overall reliability and validity are usually weak. These disadvantages can be partially dealt with by taking care to avoid bias on the part of the interviewer, respondent and question content. Interviewers may misinterpret and respondents may not answer the question honestly, gearing responses to what they think the interviewer may want them to say.

Within the interview process responses need to be recorded. The taking of notes, however, is likely to break the continuity of the interaction. While audio tapes are useful, there is potential for problems with transcription. However, whilst it is essential to consider all the possible problems, conducting semi-structured interviews allows for assessing meaning and understanding. This type of interview has a more personal approach, is flexible and adaptable, allowing for in-depth discussion. An interview encourages rapport and places minimal restraint on the respondent's answers (Cohen and Manion, 1985).

Designing and constructing an interview schedule requires the same care and attention as that given to the questionnaire. Furthermore, the interview is an alternative and complementary method to the questionnaire. As Valentine (1982) remarks, the problems raised by taking introspective reports are no more serious than the problems raised by other methods. In fact, no one method of collecting data is faultless.

The values identification grid

The values grid is a modification of Kelly's (1955) original repertory grid technique. The repertory grid offers a method of exploring the ways in which a person categorises other persons, objects or ideas. To understand a person, then one must see how he or she constructs a situation (phenomenological approach). For the purpose of the audit, the grid was modified to categorise and identify personal and organisational values. Bannister (1977) claims that constructs (in this case, values such as openness and honesty) are not just verbal labels. A controversial issue is whether the constructs should be elicited from or provided for the individual. In using the values identification grid (VIG) some organisational values had already been identified through the questionnaires and interviews but respondents were encouraged to elicit at least two of their own.

The advantage of the VIG lies in the fact that it provides an abundance of rich data open to interpretation and, to some extent, statistical analysis.

Case studies and action research

The first ethics and values audit process utilised an 'ethics hotline'. As a result of this process case studies emerged. Individual anonymity was safeguarded and confidentiality respected. For the purpose of carrying out the audit, the case studies were analysed in a similar way to the interviews as they yielded a thematic source of data relating to ethical issues and values within the organisation.

The case study method also complements aspects of action research. Hasley (1972) remarks that action research involves small-scale intervention, involvement and participation within the real world and a close examination of the effects of that intervention. It is participatory in the sense that the team is directly involved in the research and acts upon the problem presented through a case study approach. According to Cohen and Manion (1985), the principal aims of action research are to improve practice.

Analysis of policies

Information was obtained from a number of groups within the organisation in relation to existing policies. This information, together with a selective analysis of existing policies and charters, was linked to data derived from the questionnaires, values grids, interviews and case studies.

Summary

The methods discussed were used in carrying out the first EVA and yielded a rich source of data and material. In spite of some limitations, each method complements others and allows for inference and interpretation (Cohen and Manion, 1985). However, whilst the use of several methods is important, other ways of assessing values may be considered. There will always be some restrictions on methods chosen or used, often because of limited resources. It is also essential to remember that developing a profile of organisational values is only the beginning of an ongoing process for developing an ethical system for managing change. Wilson (1993b), in his paper on the role of research in business ethics, sets out a model for action which describes how research may influence managers and organisations. He states that research may move managers and organisations from a position of talking about business ethics to actually implementing ethical working practices. Wilson rightly remarks that organisations may stop with the production of a code of ethics or perhaps a charter. The danger is that if the process stops at this point, the code or charter may sit on shelves gathering dust. According to Wilson values ought to be translated into business actions. Wilson's model of action includes ethics as an important part of training, recruitment, selection, promotion and pay and reward systems. He also encourages conducting an ethics audit, processes that deal with unethical behaviour, establishing values, developing codes and setting up ethics committees. These issues are discussed in detail in Chapter 9 and clearly parallel the ongoing process and outcome of the EVA.

References

Bannister, D. (1977) *A Manual for RepGrid Techniques*. Academic Press, London.

Bellah, R.N., Madsen, R., Sullivan, W.M., Swidler, A. and Tipton, S.M. (1988) *Habits of the Heart: Individualism and Commitment in American Life*. Harper & Row, New York.

Cohen, L. and Manion, L. (1985) *Research Methods in Education*. Croom Helm, London.

Hasley, A.H. (1972) *Educational Priority: Problems and Policies*. HMSO, London.

Henry, C., Drew, J., Anwar, N., Campbell, G. and Benoit-Asselman, D. (1992) *EVA Project: The Ethics and Values Audit*. University of Central Lancashire, Preston.

Kelly, G. (1955) *The Psychology of Personal Constructs*. Norton, New York.

Macleod Clark, J. and Hockey, L. (1989) *Further Research in Nursing*. Scutari Press, London.

Nesbit, J.D. and Entwistle, N.J. (1970) *Educational Research Methods*. University of London Press, London.

Valentine, E.R. (1982) *Conceptual Issues in Psychology*. Allen and Unwin, London.

Wall, A. (1993) *Values and the NHS: A Briefing Paper*. Institute of Health Services Management, London.

White, P. (1987) *Self-respect, Self-esteem and the Management of Educational Institutions: A Question of Values in Educational Management and Administration*, **15**, 85–91.

Wilcox, J. and Ebbs, S. (1992) *The Leadership Compass: Values in Higher Education*. George Washington University, Washington DC.

Wilson, A. (1993a) Translating corporate values into business behaviour. *Journal of Business Ethics: A European Review*, **2(2)**, 103–5.

Wilson, A. (1993b) *Getting Ethics on the Business Agenda – The Role of Research*. The British Academy of Management Annual Conference, Milton Keynes.

Appendix 2 A summary of the EVA Report

Jane Pritchard

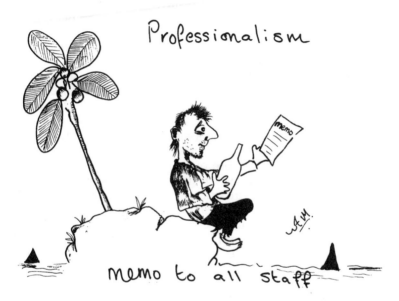

Preface

Ever since 1986, when Lancashire Polytechnic (now known as the University of Central Lancashire) became the first higher education institution in the UK to adopt a mission statement, it had been an institution which claimed widespread commitment to an agreed purpose. The first sentence of the mission statement committed the University to 'encourage and enable individuals to develop their full potential'. The frequency of reference to the mission statement in University documents and by University management was striking but how far had the values underlying the mission statement really permeated the University? In 1992, the University of Central Lancashire commissioned a team (consisting of five seconded staff of the institution and led by Professor Christine Henry) to conduct an ethics and values audit. The team conducted a large number of interviews and administered questionnaires throughout the institution in an endeavour not only to research the ethics and values of the University and its staff, but also to try to answer the question 'Does the University practise what it preaches?'. In line with the policy of openness of the University, the findings and recommendations arising from the audit were widely circulated. The audit report revealed strengths and weaknesses in the University and whilst, not unexpectedly, the media concentrated on the latter, the debate which followed in the institution was far more balanced and helped the University to come to terms with the need to continue to develop all of its practices if its mission statement was to become a reality.

In this appendix, Jane Pritchard summarises the report of the audit in a manner which seeks to show the benefits and difficulties of the process for other organisations. This preface attempts to put the report into the context of the era in which it took place.

In 1992, the University had just come through several years of very rapid change and had every reason to expect this period of change to continue. Prior to 1988, the University (then Lancashire Polytechnic) had, like other polytechnics, been under the legal control of its local education authority (Lancashire). Under the local authority, the institution had grown quickly and developed a clear mission which had driven its activities. However, in 1988, the pace of change accelerated sharply. The government passed legislation which made each polytechnic an independent corporation. A new board was appointed at incorporation of Lancashire Polytechnic on 1 April 1989 and a new rector (the prevalent title in Europe for the post more usually described in England as the vice chancellor) took over in the autumn of 1989. A new faculty and departmental system was introduced in 1990. A five year strategic plan was agreed in 1988 which would see the number of students at the University double in the period of the plan. Simultaneously, the University academic board decided to introduce a credit accumulation and transfer scheme (CATS) thus committing the University to a complete reconsideration and conversion of its curriculum. To achieve the rapid growth in the number of students required, the opportunity was taken to introduce a significant number of new courses, which the staff needed to develop and have validated via the delegated powers which the then Polytechnic had received from the Council for National Academic Awards (CNAA) and later via the University's own powers to award degrees and higher degrees as from September 1992. A network of partner institutions had been established locally, regionally and internationally to facilitate access to the University and opportunities for exchange. A large number of new staff were appointed in a short period of time, so that, by 1992, half the staff of the University had been in post for under three years. All these changes were taking place whilst the government was squeezing the funding in higher education so that the growth in income of the University lagged behind the growth in students. Few expected that when Lancashire Polytechnic joined the new unified sector of higher education as the University of

Central Lancashire, it would lead to increased funding in real terms. In these circumstances, some staff felt that the pressures on them, which had grown throughout the last five years, would continue to mount.

The world of the University of Central Lancashire was changing fast and it was inevitable that many of its members felt that they were at best reacting to, rather than controlling, those changes. Although by any external or comparative analysis, the institution was being extremely successful, it was clear that not all staff felt empowered by this success.

In this situation, the management of the University was convinced that there remained a high level of commitment among staff and considerable evidence of widespread shared values. It recognised, however, that many staff did not feel valued and that some had lost faith in some aspects of the way in which the University was being managed. In these circumstances, rather than falling back on blaming problems on 'poor communication', the decision was taken to conduct an ethics and values audit and so to air any problems which might exist. It was recognised that this was a risky strategy in that, once given terms of reference, the audit team would be free to follow the issues and produce a publicly available report. However, having had an openness policy for several years, this was not an unfamiliar situation in which to be placed!

The audit was duly conducted and its report widely circulated. There followed a period of debate in which the University came to terms with the findings of the report and the members of the University (including the management) developed their understanding of the paramount importance of good interpersonal relationships, clear communication, professional behaviour and ethical standards.

It is still too early to say how much the audit led to changes at the University but I can see how it changed the behaviour of myself and colleagues. Accountability and openness grew as did a recognition that each member of the University community has a responsibility not only to behave fairly to other members but also to be prepared to explain one's actions. The audit process itself and the willingness of the University management to risk exposure by commissioning the audit were also significant. Anyone involved in management may be tempted to feel that there is enough criticism voiced without commissioning more, but unless an organisation can recognise and respond to the feelings of its members, its future will be limited. It is certainly the view of the University of Central Lancashire, on the basis of the experience since 1992, that an ethics and values audit can make a worthwhile contribution to the process of organisational self-understanding. In a rapidly changing world, such self-understanding is a prerequisite for future success.

Alan Roff
Vice Rector
January 1994

Introduction

This summary is intended to provide a brief insight into the full EVA Report published in 1992. The Ethics and Values Audit (EVA) project was commissioned by the University of Central Lancashire as an internal investigation of its own practices. By reference to various research methods including a confidential questionnaire sent to staff at all levels, the project sought to assess its performance in practice by reference to its own mission statement. The EVA Report sets out to answer the question 'Does the University practise what it preaches?'

As the whole Report is expressed as being based on the mission statement this document is reproduced in full at the beginning of this summary.

The original EVA Report was essentially an in-house investigation into the university's own operation. Since publication there has been considerable interest in the report and particularly in the applicability of the audit process to other organisations.

Whilst this summary intends to adhere to the integrity of the report any variations are made to change the emphasis from looking inwards at the university's own operation to looking outwards to a more general application in order to stress the transferability of the audit process to other institutions and corporate structures. If such transferability is not emphasised in the original report it is certainly implicit.

Layout of Report

Divided into three sections, the first part gives a full commentary on the research methods and results culminating with the research team's recommendations for ensuring the practical realisation of the commitments made by the University's mission statement. The second part consists of an analysis of the data obtained through the research methods. The final part of the report identifies the external context of the report and includes a profile of the research team.

The audit team

Christine Henry has a professional background in health, psychology and education. Her academic development and interests are in the areas of philosophy, ethics and psychology specifically related to the professional fields of education, health and management.

Janine Drew has a professional background in diverse areas of administration. Her academic development and interests are in English literature, applied philosophy and ethics and management practice within organisations.

Naseem Anwar has a professional background in the wide area of equal opportunities. His academic development and interests are in social science and applied ethics in both the health and social areas.

George Campbell has a professional background in education. His academic development and interests are in English, cultural studies and applied ethics in higher education.

David Benoit-Asselman has a professional background in administration and courses review. His academic development and interests are in philosophy, counselling and ethics in education.

Louise Williams has been the unit's personal assistant. She has a background in office administration and her interests are in professional administration.

Background and context to the Report

The mission statement and other management documents referred to in the report:

> . . . indicate a dynamism in the organisation because of the focus on important organisational values. They provide the theory behind the statement: 'The University of Central Lancashire is a caring place.' But is this really the case? Some would say no, and suggest that there are times of dramatic change in higher education where competition is the real value. In effect there appears to be a double standard: one value is preached, caring, and another is practised, competition.
>
> (The EVA Report, p1)

To investigate the truth or otherwise of this statement was the task of the audit team. The last years have seen great changes in higher education. It can be argued that the ethos has changed from providing education in an atmosphere of quiet and untimed learning to operating a business where the student is the customer and the degree course is the product.

Such change is not confined to Higher Education. Almost every sector of our society is affected by an ever-increasing requirement to give account for cost and to give 'value' for money. There is a danger that at such times an organisation's most important resource, its human resource, can be obscured. The Report implies that this can be a result of short-term policies and knee-jerk reactions to new and crisis situations; quick solutions that fail to give proper regard to the long-term commitments set out in, for example, a mission statement. By adhering to the provisions of well constructed and relevant codes of practice and ethical conduct organisations can safeguard themselves against the pitfalls of crisis management in times of change.

The process of identifying and exploring values involves research, analysis, debate and discovering ways of enhancing ethical practice within the organisation. Organisations can enhance their professional standing by presenting a high ethical profile and adhering to the best codes of practice available. By carrying out the EVA project, a further step has been taken towards quality enhancement. In one sense, this means caring for 'human resources' and this in turn will enhance quality. It is the beginning of a journey of never ending improvement.

(The EVA Report, 1992, p2)

Guidelines to Terminology

Principles	are guidelines for human conduct. They have a broad or universal application and may be seen as fundamental to the way in which we behave towards each other. For example *'Treat others as you would wish to be treated yourself'* – from this arises respect for others as persons.
Values	are much broader than principles and may not necessarily be moral; for example, a gang of thieves may share values. However, moral values are like maps that arise from our experiences and have a subjective interpretation. Values can support or violate principles.
Ethics	assess the ways in which we behave and the quality of moral values that we have. Ethics offers a way of enquiring into our behaviour and moral justification for actions and choices. The use of ethical theories may help to resolve conflict between alternative options.
Professional ethics	derives from ethics in that it is applied to professional practice. It considers the way in which professionals practise and encourage guidelines for codes of professional conduct. Professional ethics also deal with ethical concerns related to the power, role and position of professionals. For example, maintaining confidentiality between doctor and patient or solicitor and client.
Morals	This term in everyday language is used to mean the same as ethics. Morals concern human conduct and values, whereas ethics is the study of both.

The following sections have the same headings as the EVA Report but summarise the contents of the relevant sections. Again, any departure from a faithful rendering is to stress the applicability to organisations other than the University of Central Lancashire of what is said and also, of course, for ease of reading in this much shorter form.

Themes

The themes give an overall profile of ethics and values within the University.

(EVA Report, 1992, p6)

The report identifies ten themes as emerging from the investigation. The emphasis is on communication, interpersonal relationships and the priorities behind the distribution of resources. The importance of these issues is, of course, their consequential effect on staff morale. Where there is a lack of official (managerial) dissemination of appropriate and essential information coupled with a lack of consultation in decision making, staff feel unvalued. The resultant reduction in motivation could have serious consequences for the effectiveness of any organisation.

There is a well-developed informal network of collaboration and communication amongst staff that acknowledges the importance of openness, honesty and trust. The Report rather implies that such a system has developed for want of a more orthodox network.

The final theme reports dissatisfaction with the amount of time and resources made available for research and spending with students.

Two quotations from the research are set out:

'They just pack them in and teach them and they haven't got time for research'.

'It's [the organisation] very task oriented, it doesn't take account of people'.

Organisational perspectives

An organisation is structurally an entity in itself. Certain values can be imposed upon it in terms of its public image and explicitly stated goals and objectives. However, the organisation is also a reflection of the beliefs and values of the individuals within it. The two sets of value systems may not always be the same.

(EVA Report, 1992, p8)

Values and goals shared by the organisation and the individuals that comprise it are identified as an essential feature of an organisation's success. An individual will work hard for an organisation that values his/her contribution. The Report states that the relationship between an individual and an organisation depends not only on the terms and conditions of a legal contract of employment but also on the psychological contract that underlies it. Such a psychological contract deals with issues of self-worth, future expectation, loyalty and respect. Breaches of the psychological contract can cause emotional responses that can lead to, perhaps, irrational reactions that can be diverted to 'unreasonable' attitudes regarding aspects of the legal contract, for example, an unrealistic emphasis on pay and working conditions. In turn this can lead to the organisation misunderstanding the priorities of its employees.

Generally the fact that the organisation commissioned the Audit into values and ethics did much to reassure staff that values such as openness, collaboration, respect, responsibility and morality were important to the organisation and that there was room for these as well as clear concern for profitability and competition. Where an organisation is undergoing rapid change the Report identifies that such issues must be kept to the forefront of the organisation's considerations. Otherwise there is a real danger that there will be depressed motivation and morale, poor decision making and conflict leading to lack of co-operation.

Communication

The Report finds some evidence of poor communication. This is seen as being at least partly due to the complex hierarchical structure of the organisation resulting in inconsistent passing of information between the layers.

> When the official communication network does not operate effectively, individuals find an alternative information network based on rumour and often wrong assumptions. This can be highly divisive and often leads to unnecessary conflicts.
>
> (EVA Report, 1992, p11)

Participation

There are two marked views towards staff relations that are contrasted. The first regards employees as being primarily motivated by money. The aspirations of individuals are likely to be very different from those of the organisation and staff must therefore be 'controlled'.

The other view, whilst recognising the importance of reasonable remuneration, believes that, as well, employees are strongly motivated by there being meaning and satisfaction in their work. Clearly the two points of view lead to very different styles of management. The one will put its trust in a strong hierarchical structure whilst the other will see its interest promoted by close consultation and collaboration to ensure that an agreed programme can be formulated which synthesises the aims of both the employees and the organisation.

Resources and research and advanced study

The Report acknowledges the achievement of the University in remaining financially stable in times of extreme economic struggle. It points out, however, that the research reveals some dissatisfaction from staff members about the allocation of resources. Staff members feel that more time and money should be given to individual students and research.

> I do not think education can proceed at a higher level without research.
>
> (A quotation from the questionnaires)

No manager will be unfamiliar with staff dissatisfaction about the prioritising of resources. What is remarkable, however, is the implication that the distribution of assets, if not condoned, would be better understood with a greater involvement of staff in the decision process.

Management style and organisational practices

> A theme that has consistently arisen through the Audit data is a concern with inappropriate styles of management and management practices.
>
> (EVA Report, p14)

The Report identifies which styles of management form an important constituent to the 'culture' of an organisation. It centres on five aspects:

1. *Reporting Mechanisms.* There is revealed a degree of cynicism throughout the organisation as to the presence of trust, openness and honesty in the dissemination of information.

2. *Problems and Conflicts.* Rather than a spirit of 'all working together' there is some evidence of interdepartmental and even interpersonal rivalry giving rise to a distortion of the motives used in decision making.

3. *Applications of Procedures and Regulations*. Evidence of inconsistent application of rules and regulations can lead to frustration and a sense of injustice.

4. *Organisational Policies*. The Report reveals a belief that there is inconsistency between the University's public and private acts. This leaves the organisation open to the suggestion of a lack of integrity.

5. *Use and Abuse of Power and Role*. The Report reveals some evidence that individuals who learn to 'play the system' receive favour whereas those who do not feel marginalised. This feature is described as being a common characteristic of strongly hierarchical structures. It implies that 'vying for personal favour' is open to abuse. The power games that ensue can distort the University's true endeavour.

Climate

A great variety of personal perspectives have emerged from the investigation. Also, viewpoints have been expressed by various groups within the University. For example, separate views were sought from students and from staff, both clerical and academic. Whilst many views refer to positive features of University life, for example, it has put considerable energy into its policy of equal opportunities and reducing sexual harassment, a common view emerges that the University fails properly to value the individual. This is ascribed in part to the very rapid growth of the organisation in recent years and partly to an overly authoritarian style of management. This leads to a lack of openness to new ideas suggested by individuals, a feeling of lack of personal autonomy and a lack of respect for each other. The dominant style of management is not confined to the administration but in some instances is reported to have carried over into relations between lecturers and students. One quotation from a questionnaire reports:

> sometimes students . . . have been patronised or ridiculed or whatever by members of staff . . .

Values in the curriculum

The EVA Report acknowledges that it has been unable to carry out a thorough examination of the University's curriculum within the constraints of the time and accessibility of information available. The brief insight recorded shows some evidence of ethical considerations being present. Suffice it to say that this might be an area of further study.

Policy analysis

Implicit throughout this summary is the Report's analysis of policy at the University of Central Lancashire. It is not necessary for this summary to set it out again. The University's commitment to finding ways of improving its ethical profile commenced with the commission of the Report. The spirit is embodied in a quotation from Lord Milner set out in the EVA Report (p28):

> If we believe a thing to be bad, and if we have a right to prevent it, it is our duty to try and prevent it and to damn the consequences.

Methodology

The whole of Part Two of the EVA Report is devoted to a detailed description of the material obtained through the various research methods. The material is presented in a variety of ways: tables, grids, graphs and the like. It is not appropriate for this summary to discuss the fine detail of the findings of the audit team. Its purpose is best served by stating the general principles of the audit process. The function of this summary is not to delve into the peculiarities of the University of Central Lancashire but to illustrate the relevance of the endeavour to *organisations of all kinds,* particularly those employing the services of large numbers of professionals, by reference to the University's experience.

Anyone wanting to know in more detail how the audit was carried out and what methods of investigation were used must be referred to the original Report or, for a more personal explanation, to the Centre for Professional Ethics based at the University which has grown out of the EVA Project.

The final section of the Report deals with more detailed definitions of terminology used by the Report, gives a comprehensive bibliography of source and general reading surrounding the Project and adds some more detailed information to the University's policies, for example that for equal opportunities and ethics. It contains a report from the students' union that repeats the Report's own acknowledgement that there is scope for further study into the position and standpoint of the student body.

The foreword to the Report is given by Dr John R. Wilcox, who is a Director of a Centre for Professional Ethics in America, and Part Three of the Report includes a tribute to the work carried out by him in this area as portrayed in *The Leadership Compass: Values and Ethics in Higher Education* written in 1992 by himself and Dr Susan L. Ebbs.

There is one section in Part One of the Report that has not yet been dealt with in this Summary, namely the section dealing with the

Report's recommendations. Before concluding it is essential that these should now be mentioned.

Recommendations of the EVA Report

> They represent an attempt to encourage a University management style and culture in which recognition of and respect for all members of its community is the paramount value and where a climate of genuine trust, participation in decision-making and collaboration is fostered. The assumption then is that good and fair ethical practice will naturally evolve and become the norm.
>
> (EVA Report, p32)

This statement embodies the recommendations of the Report. Fourteen factors are identified.

1. *University leadership*. More personal involvement is requested by management. Staff feelings of not counting or being undervalued would be reduced if there was more face to face contact between staff and senior managers.

2. *Management style*. More consultation is advocated with a greater flow of information, going 'upwards' as well as 'downwards.' A well-debated charter for management is seen as a very positive advancement coupled, of course, to the subsequent adherence to the ethical principles thereof.

3. *Organisational culture*. Again a greater degree of collaboration is stressed with a higher leadership profile present which encourages a more caring culture.

4. *The mission statement*. This should be continually reviewed to ensure that it honestly reflects the beliefs of all the members of the University. Once agreed, every effort should be made to fulfil its commitments.

5. *Code of professional practice*. It is recommended that a code should be developed and adopted. Clearly a code can deal with more practical detail than is appropriate for a mission statement.

6. *The establishment of a director* with particular responsibility for human resources and internal communications. This is felt to manifest a true commitment to a person centred approach to management. This post would be responsible for putting into practice the recommendations of the Report.

7. *Internal secondment of a human resource and internal communications co-ordinator*. Such a person would assist the Director when appointed and provide 'local knowledge'.

8. *Staff handbook*. As well as the more usual contents of such a document the Report sees this as an important vehicle for giving advice about ethical issues with practical examples of how to act in common situations.

9. *Continued improvements of the working environment and creation of common staff space*. This enables physical endorsement to be given to the principle of good communication.

10. *Development of a cross-university 'learning' community*. Workshops and similar forums should be encouraged for discussion both internally and with other similar organisations. This will encourage thought and fresh ideas.

11. *Ethics and values audit for students*. It has already been stated that a need for such an audit is acknowledged.

12. *'Values' in the curriculum audit*. This, too, has already been referred to as an area of future study.

13. *Ethics and values adviser/facilitator*. This is seen as an arbitrator's role rather than that of a negotiator or counsellor.

14. *Dissemination of Report and its recommendations*. Throughout the Report has promoted respect and acknowledgement for work done. It is only fair and ethical that the same treatment should be afforded to itself! Consistent with its own recommendation for greater collaboration it asks for written responses to the Report from all departments and services and asks senior management for an urgent indication as to how, and by when, the recommendations of the Report will be implemented.

Conclusions

It could be argued that many of the techniques used by the EVA Report have been used by management consultants for many years. This may be so; the reports of such consultants have doubtless been analysed in great detail by boardrooms throughout the world. How often, however, have such reports been published and offered up for public scrutiny?

What is remarkable about the EVA Report is the brave commitment to ethical practice shown by the University of Central Lancashire; firstly, by commissioning the Report at all, but secondly, and most importantly, by its complete submission to airing its business and staff relations to the world, 'warts and all'.

Such unfearing faith in the sincerity of its pledge to change and improvement is a lesson to all. Confidential reports are so often invitations to cover up what is undesirable. Organisations that are afraid to be open must surely have something to hide. If what is to be done with the results of an investigation is not clear from the outset, employees taking part and answering questionnaires will not feel safe and will not be disposed to answer questions honestly. Clearly the cost and time spent on 'closet' enquiries will be wasted. Such exercises are exposed to accusations of 'pure veneer', at best nothing more than empty exercises of public relations, at worst underhand means of gathering information which will be used for uncertain and probably ominous ends.

The University of Central Lancashire must also be praised for establishing, as far as possible in the confines of an organisation, the Ethics Unit that carried out the audit as an independent entity. The psychological confidence that this inspired in staff taking part in the investigation is a powerful symbol of integrity in itself and truly embodies the University's commitment to ethical practice.

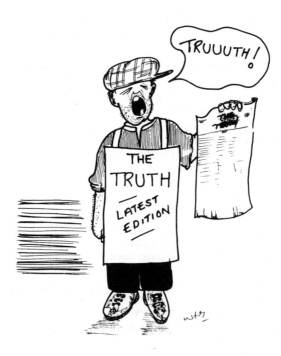

Bibliography

Abelson, R. (1977) *Persons: A Study in Philosophical Psychology*. Macmillan, London.
Apps, J. (1993) Nursing education and practice. *Journal of Advances in Health Care*, **2**, **(3)** 45–50.
Arnot, M (ed.) (1985) *Race and Gender. Equal Opportunities Policies in Education*. Pergamon Press, Oxford.
Arygris, C. (1976) *Increasing Leadership Effectiveness*. J Wiley & Sons, New York.
Balogh, R. and Beattie, A. (1988) *Performance Indicators in Nursing Education*. ENB, Sheffield.
Balogh, R. and Beattie, A. (1991) *Defining Quality in Training Institutions*, Nursing Times, **87** **(87)**, 44–7.
Beauchamp, T.L. and Childress, J.F. (1979) *Principles of Biomedical Ethics*. Oxford University Press, Oxford.
Bellah, R.N. *et al*, (1985) *Habits of the Heart: Individualism and Commitment to American Life*. Berkeley University Press, Berkeley, USA.
Bellah, R.N., Madsen, R., Sullivan, W.M., Swidler, A., Tipton, S.M. (1988), *Habits of the Heart: Individualism and Commitment in American Life*. Harper Row, New York.
Berlin, I. (1993) *Joseph de Maistre and the origins of Fascism*, in *The Crooked Timber of Humanity, Chapters in the History of Ideas*, pp.91–174. Vintage Books, Random House, New York.
Beyerstein, D. (1993) *The Functions and Limitations of Professional Codes of Ethics*. In *Applied Ethics; A Reader*, (eds) E.R. Winkler, J.R. Coombes, Blackwell Scientific Publications, Oxford.
Blane, D. (1986) *Health Professionals*. Chapter 10. In: *Sociology as applied to Medicine*, (eds) D. Patrick and G. Scanbler. Baillière & Tindall, London.
Buckle, S. (1991, 1993) *Natural Law* in *A Companion to Ethics*, P. Singer, (ed.) Blackwell Publishers, Oxford.
Byshee, J. (1990) Strength status and respect. *Nursing, The Journal of Clinical Practice, Education and Management*, **4(1)** 20–3.
Carroll, L. (1984 edn.) *Alice through the Looking Glass*. Puffin Classics, Penguin Books, London.
Chadwick, R. (1993) *Justice in Priority Setting*. In *Rationing in Action*. BMJ Publishing Group, London.
Copley, T. *et al.*, (1990) *Forms of Assessment in Religious Education. The Main Report of the FARE Project* (The FARE Project).
Cornwall Education Committee (1989) *Syllabus for Religious Education*.
Covey, S. (1989) *The Seven Habits of Highly Effective People: Restoring the Character Ethic*. Simon and Schuster, New York.
Davis, J. (1989) *Who or What are Lecturer Practitioners?* Senior Nurse 9 10 22.
De Marco, J.P., and Fox, M. (1986) *New Directions in Ethics: The Challenge of Applied Ethics*. Routledge and Kegan Paul, London.
Downie, R.S. and Calman, K.C. (1987) *Healthy Respect, Ethics in Health Care*. Faber & Faber.
English National Board (1990) *Framework for Continued Professional Education and Training for Nurses*, Project paper 3, ENB, London.
Epstein, E. (1987) Annual conference of the European Business Ethics Network.
Frederick, W., (1988) Survey Examines Corporate Ethics Policies. *Journal of Accountancy* (Feb 1988, p.16).
Fulman, M. (1982) *The Meaning of Educational Change*. Teachers College Press, New York.
Gardner, R.A., Gardner, B. and van Cantfort, T.E. (1989) *Teaching Sign Language to Chimpanzees*. State University of New York Press, New York.
Gillion, R. (1986) *Philosophical Medical Ethics*. John Wiley & Sons, London.
Gintis, H. and Bowles, S. (1981) Contradiction and Reproduction in Educational Theory. In *Education and the State* **1**, R. Dale *et al.*, (eds) Open University Press, Milton Keynes.

Growler, D. (1972) On the Concept of Being a Person, In *Six Approaches to the Person*, R. Ruddock (ed.), Manchester University Press, Manchester.

Guardian Education Supplement, 24th November (1992).

Hare, R.M. (1964) *The Language of Morals*. Oxford University Press.

Harris, J. (1991) *The Value of Life*. Routledge, London.

Harris, N.G.E. (1989) *Professional Codes of Conduct in the United Kingdom*. Mansell Publishing, London.

Henry, C. (1986) *Conceptions of the Nature of Persons*. Unpublished PhD, Leeds University.

Henry, C. (1992) Reasonable Care: Approaches to health care research. In *Journal of Advances in Health and Nursing Care* **1** (4).

Henry, C., Drew, J., Anwar, N. Campbell, G. and Benoit-Asselman, D. (1992) *The EVA Project: The Ethics and Values Audit*. University of Central Lancashire, Preston.

Henry, C. and Pashley, G. (1990) *Health Ethics*, Quay Publishers, Lancaster.

Henry, C. and Pashley, G. (1990) Carving Out the Nursing 90's, *Nursing Times*, **86 (3)**.

Heywood Jones, I. (1990) *The Nurses Code*, Macmillan, London.

HMSO (1979 & 1992) *Nurses Midwives and Health Visitors Acts*.

HMSO-Hansard (1988) *Parliamentary Debates (Hansard) House of Commons* No.130 columns 403, 411, 416.

HMSO-DHSS (1989) *A Strategy for Nursing*, DOH, London.

HMSO (1990) *NHS and Community Care Act*.

HMSO (1990) *Working for Patients. NHS Trusts: A Working Guide*.

HMSO-DES (1991) *Parent's Charter*. Department of Education and Science, London.

HMSO (1992) *The Patient's Charter*. Department of Health 51-1003-10/91 C5000.

HMSO DFE (1993) *The Charter for Higher Education*. Department for Education, London.

Jagger, A.M. (1993) *Feminist Problems and Human Nature*. Rowman & Allenhead, Harvester Press, Sussex.

Jennings, B. (1986) *Applied Ethics and the Vocation of Social Science*. In: *New Directions in Ethics* J.P. De Marco, and R.M. Fox (eds) Routledge and Kegan Paul, New York.

Jones, J. (1993) *Chimp Talk*. BBC Horizon Publication. BBC London.

Kant, I. (1984) What is Enlightenment? In *German Aesthetic and Literary Criticism; Kant, Fichte, Schelling, Schopenhaur, Hegel*, D. Simpson (ed.), CUP, Cambridge.

Kearney, A. and Diamond, J. (1990) 'Access Courses: A New Orthodoxy?' *Journal of Further and Higher Education* **14(1)**.

Kelly, C.M. (1988) *The Destructive Achiever: Power and Ethics in the American Corporation*. Addison-Wesley, New York.

Kelly, G. (1955) *The Psychology of Personal Constructs*. Norton, New York.

Kendrick, K and Simpson, A. (1992) In *Themes and Perspectives in Nursing*, K. Soothill, C. Henry and K. Kendrick (eds), Chapman and Hall, London.

Keyserlingk, E.W. (1993) Ethics Codes and Guidelines for Health Care and Research; Can Respect for Autonomy be a Multi-cultural Principle? In *Applied Ethics: A Reader*, E.R. Winkler, J.R. Coombs (eds), Blackwell Publishers, Oxford.

Komrad, M.S. (1983) A Defense of Medical Paternalism: Maintaining Patient Autonomy. *Journal of Medical Ethics* **9**, Blackwell Publishers, Oxford.

Kuhlman, S. and Jones, M. (1991) *Managing Radical Change*, MHNA.

Law Society, The (1974) *A Guide to the Professional Conduct of Solicitors*, The Law Society, London.

Locke, John (1964 edn.) Book III, Of Words. *An Essay Concerning Human Understanding. 1690*. Everyman, Dent, London.

Loveridge, R. and Starkey, K. (eds) (1992) *Continuity and Crisis in the NHS*. Open University Press, Buckingham.

MacFarlane, B. (1992) 'The Thatcherite' Generation and University Degree Results', *Journal of Further and Higher Education* **16(22)**.

MacIntyre, A. (1981) *After Virtue*. Duckworth, London.

McInerney, P. (1992) *Introduction to Philosophy*. Harper Perennial, New York.

Midgley, M. (1991) *Wisdom, Information and Wonder*. Routledge, London.

Moloney, M. (1993) *Professionalization in Nursing, Current Trends and Issues*. Lippincott, London.

Neal, D. (ed.) (1982) *Spirituality Across the Curriculum*. College of St Mark & St John Foundation, Plymouth.

NFER (1991) *NFER Project 2000 Research, Interim Paper 3*. NFER, Slough.

Norman, R. (1983) *The Moral Philosophers*. Oxford University Press, Oxford.

Nuttall J. (1993) *Moral Questions, an Introduction to Ethics*. Polity Press and Blackwell, Cambridge.

Observer, The. Article, November 7 1993.

Ong, W.J. (1982) *Orality and Literacy*. Methuen, London.

Osmond, R. (1993) *Changing Perspectives, Christian Culture and Morals in England Today*. Darton, Longman & Todd, London.

Plato (1990 edn.) *Euryphro*. In *Classics of Western Philosophy*, S.D. Cahn (ed.) Hackett, Indianapolis/Cambridge.

Pritchard, J. (1993) *Charters, Charters and More Charters!* Paper, International Conference on Professional and Business Ethics, University of Central Lancashire, October 1993.

Procter, S. and Reed, J. (1993) *Nurse Education – A Reflective Approach*. Edward Arnold, London.

Raiborn, C.A. and Payne, D. (1990) Corporate Codes of Conduct: A Collective Conscience and Continuum, *Journal of Business Ethics*, 9:879–889. Kluwer Academic Publishers, Netherlands.

Reeves, M. (1988) *The Crisis in Higher Education: Competence, Delight and the Common Good*. Open University Press, Milton Keynes.

Royal College of Nursing (1993) *Teaching in a Different World*. An RCN discussion document.

Ruggiero, V.R. (1973) *The Moral Imperative*. Alfred Publishers, New York.

Saussure, F. (1992) A General Course on Linguistics. In *A Critical and Cultural Reader*, A. Easthope, and K. McGowan (eds). Open University Press, Buckingham.

Scheffler, I. (1985) *Of Human Potential: An essay in the Philosophy of Education*. Routledge and Kegan Paul, London.

Shaw, W.H. and Barry, V. (1992) *Moral Issues in Business*. Wadsworth, California.

Sikora, R.I. (1993) *Rule-Utilitarianism and Applied Ethics*. In *Applied Ethics*, E.R. Winkler, and J.C. Coombs (eds) Blackwell Publishers, Oxford.

Snoeyenbos, M. and Jewell, D. (eds: M. Snoeyenbos, R. Almeder, and J. Humber) (1983) *Morals, Management and Codes in Business Ethics*. Buffalo, New York.

Soothill, K., Henry, C., and Kendrick, K. (eds) (1992) *Themes and Perspectives in Nursing*. Chapman & Hall, London.

Stern, K. (1993) Court Ordered Caesarean Sections. *The Modern Law Review* **56 (2)** 238–43.

Stone, C.D. (1975) *Where the Law Ends*. Harper Row, New York.

Straw, J. (1989) *Equal Opportunities: The Way Ahead*. Institute of Personnel Management, London.

Thompson, J.L. (1990) *Strategic Management*. Chapman & Hall, London.

Tierney, W.G. (1988) Organisational Culture in Higher Education: Defining the Essentials *Journal of Higher Education* **59 (1)**, 2–21. Ohio State University Press.

Warnock, M. (1985) *A Question of Life*. Blackwell Publishers, Oxford.

Watts, G. (1992) Implementing Project 2000: The Need for Evaluation and Review. In *Project 2000*, O. Slevin, and M. Buckenham (eds) Campion Press, Edinburgh.

White, P. (1987) *Self-respect, Self-esteem and the Management of Educational Institutions: A Question of Values in Educational Management and Administration* **15** 85–91. British Educational Management and Administration Society.

Wilcox, J.R. and Ebbs, S.L. (1992) *The Leadership Compass: Values and Ethics in Higher Education*. George Washington University, Washington DC.

Wilcox, J.R. and Ebbs, S.L. (1992) Promoting an Ethical Climate on Campus: The Values Audit. *NASPA Journal* **29(4):** 253–60.

Williams, B. (1985) *Ethics and the Limits of Philosophy*. Harvard University Press, Cambridge, Mass.

Wilson, A. (1993) Translating Corporate Values into Business Behaviour. *A European Review* **2 (2)** April 103–5.

Wilson, A. (1993) *Getting Ethics on the Business Agenda – The Role of Research*. The British Academy of Management Annual Conference, Milton Keynes.

Index